MY HOOMAN AND ME

A Dog's Story From Street To Medical Miracle

MY HOOMAN AND ME

by

Barbara A. Mudge

...and Cassie

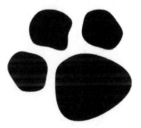

MY HOOMAN AND ME
A Dog's Story From Street
To Medical Miracle

FIRST EDITION
Copyright © 2022 by Barbara A. Mudge
Registration Number: TXu 2-336-958

International Standard Book Number: 979-8-9871385-0-2

BarbaraAMudgePublishing
Cathedral City, California USA

Book & cover design: Barbara A. Mudge
Used with permission:
"Angel" original oil by Chuck Caplinger

Printed in the United States of America

DEDICATION

With appreciation, I dedicate the telling of our story to the millions of pet rescuers who open their homes to give our loving animals the life they deserve.

Your sacrifice and care, as well as those who selflessly help get our babies to you, can be read in the eyes of our creatures whose only wish is to share with us their purity of affection.

As "hoomans" gifted with this special connection, may we continue our passion to Adopt. Don't Shop.

Acknowledgements

My thanks go out to the wonderful organization Learning In Retirement of Palm Desert, California especially the two volunteer instructors, Chris Considine and John Murrow plus my fellow classmates for taking me out of my head and providing encouragement during our memoir writing gatherings. You inspired my discipline and provided a welcome home in which to express Cassie's and my story.

I am so very grateful to my early reader, Patti Greaney for her patient third eye and for putting up with my many, many rewrites. Her feedback provided me with a much needed confidence to continue. Thanks as well go out to my friends, Bob and Yuko Jones whose friendship served as a welcome diversion, be it over pancakes or an evening of chance.

I am beholden to my spiritual upbringing which aroused this dedication to put pen to paper. With the Grace of God, our odyssey of Faith, Hope and Love resulted in a wonderful conclusion. So perfectly told in the parable of Luke 15: 3-7 "Rejoice with me, I have found my sheep that was lost," my writing was driven, perhaps, to honor His Words which so parallels our story.

Lastly, the obligation Cassie and I have to the triumvirate of lady doctors, Dr. Alexis Rambaud, DVM, Prof. Elizabeth Murchison and Dr. Maria Veronica Brignone for their devotion will remain in our hearts forever. The alliance they formed was no match for Cassie's stubborn cancer. I like to think that we got together at just the right time to attack it head-on. With hopeful optimism, my prayers are that the research on Cassie's tissues being conducted by the Transmissible Cancer Group at the Department of Veterinarian Medicine, University of Cambridge, United Kingdom will bring about an end to suffering throughout the world.

-------- Barbara

CHAPTERS

Prologue

I had fun with other dogs when I was a puppy. I sniffed their butts and let them sniff mine. We would roll around in play, chase each other down the crowded streets and hunt through the trash in the alleys. We found food behind hooman buildings - the ones with the good smells. Sometimes hoomans shooed us away but our pack leaders always found another place with yummy scents. It was okay when the big guys got all snarly with each other 'cause that's when I could grab a big bite for myself and run away from their silliness. I was a smart girl and I knew my place in the pack.

One day a boy dog jumped on me. He wasn't being silly. Afterwards my backside felt different and it hurt down there. Licking didn't make it better. It tasted and smelled funny. From then on, I tried to stay away from the pack but they were good at finding food so I followed them from the shadows. I wanted to sleep a lot but it hurt to lay down on the hard sidewalk because my skin was getting crusty and now my puppy fur was gray. When I moved, sometimes my skin split open. The goo from the cracks tasted funny too. I found an empty lot with a patch of sand – warm from the sun - and I laid down.

Alone and hungry on my patch of sand, I heard my pack barking and playing in the distance and I could smell a little bit the hooman food they found. I wanted to play too but I was so tired I couldn't move and the bump below my butt hurt me. Maybe after sleep the morning sun will help me get up and find them… and eat with them… and play with them. But tonight, I only want to sleep….

I had a new pack when I woke with the sun. There was a hooman jefa *who filled our bellies and walked me to a place that made my butt hurt go away and my fur grow shiny again. When I felt good like before other hoomans took me on a grand adventure.*

That was when I met the bestest Hooman in whose arms I felt special. She took me to a place that smelled yummy all the time and had many soft beds. She gave me toys that squeak and a big bright yard to be happy in. I felt like a puppy again and My Hooman tasted like love. I knew that this was my fur-ever home.

Then I started feeling bad again… down there… just like before. Tho My Hooman put tiny little foods down my throat that made me feel a little better, the hurting wouldn't stop. But I was with My Hooman so I didn't need to look for shadows. We went on adventures and sometimes she took me into little white rooms where our hooman pack became many. I liked how their mouths crinkled upward so I let them touch me. At home, My Hooman's warm eyes told me, "You're special, Cassie."

My journey from street to sofa to science was not easy. And what happened to me along the way is not my story alone.

This is the story of My Hooman And Me.

BIG BROWN EYES

It's said you never forget your first love.

Growing up in rural Missouri our family had many animals and although we didn't live on a farm, we lived among them: cows and chickens and frogs and snakes (for which we learned a healthy respect,) cats and dogs with whom we played and dressed up and cuddled and slept. Never caged and seldom leashed, our critter companions roamed the one-acre grounds and beyond as freely as we humans did, but like us they knew to come home where the food was.

When I was a dark-haired girl of five years, Dad brought home a bruiser of a dog named General. "He keeps jumping a neighbor's fence," Dad told us, so we took him in. "He'll make a good watch dog." I couldn't help but agree with Dad 'cause he sure as hell scared me! General, a boxer with cropped ears and a natural tail, wasn't really tall so much as hulking. But to me, that was huge especially compared to our little black mutt, "Lady." His fawn color showed well a muscular structure. Technically, Boxers are a medium-sized breed so I guess he tipped the scales on the higher end.... or maybe not. Memory doesn't serve and my perspective was that of a five-year old. My siblings played with General and Dad doted on him. Years later Mom told me she was relieved to have some added security during long days alone so far out from town with only a passel of not-yet-even-teenaged kids until Dad got home after dark. But I kept my distance from General, skeptical about my safety.

He'd have none of my aloofness, however. One day I climbed up on the kitchen booth-style banquette expecting some lunch I suppose and General hopped up right behind me. As he approached, we were eye-to-eye. Burned in my memory clearly to this day as if it were yesterday, I saw two big brown eyes filled with gentleness... filled with love. My fears of being devoured were at once replaced with a lifelong affection. There and then, sitting next to a newly devoted friend, my preference became big dogs... and, of course, only Boxers.

I don't recall many specifics about playing with General. My memories are more a feeling. I've searched but we have no family photos with him: only a quick clip on one of Dad's ubiquitous holiday home movies of General bounding behind me out the back door of our brick house as I pranced to-ward the camera in my silly Halloween costume. It's obvious on those grainy frames that he was *my* dog.

As our family aged, we eventually moved to California and had more family dogs but never another Boxer. Perhaps those suburban properties couldn't accommodate this highly energetic breed... or perhaps the last sight of General's mangled body lying on old Highway 94 was too much sadness to risk repeat.

General so loved chasing cars....

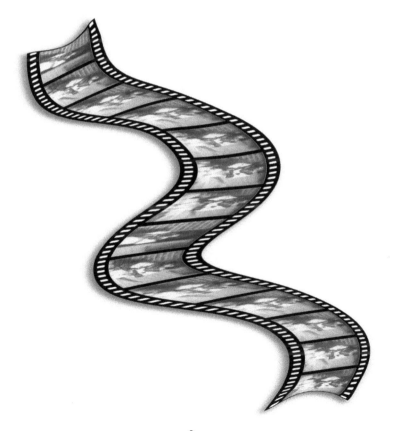

WHAT-A-BABY-GOT?

"What-a-baby-want?" starts our play sessions. Tossing the nearest stuffed toy across the backyard, I yell this baby-talk and Cassie gives chase. "Dat-a-baby-got!" I holler when she catches it. Bounding back to me, her cute little hop skip prance resembles a deer: a stubby, tiger striped, 'pocket boxer' sized deer with her full-length tail flying behind. This game of catch is different from many other dogs. It's decidedly one-sided.

Iron jaw clamped firmly around the toy, Cassie does not give up that stuffy-prey easily. "What-a-mommie-want?" I taunt as I try to pry the toy from her mouth, her whole body wiggling joyfully with resistance. Those shining eyes from behind the fluffy toy tease me with a look saying "Good luck, Mommie" as I do my best to

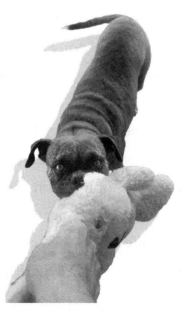

5

take back the toy and avoid a punctured finger. I succeed and our game of catch proceeds, again and again. Once sated, Cassie plops down on a nearby couch, sheltering her prey from me. "What-a-baby-got?" I ask, ending our romp. We've created our own patter, Cassie and I, as surely as any bonded couple.

I relish these play sessions because only a short time ago, Cassie's illness-wracked little body couldn't get up from the bed despite all my prompting to *Go get, go get, go get* the toy I just tossed.

Cassie and I met on Facebook. The rescue group page photo presented her, toy in mouth on a bed next to a Weimaraner. *Ooooh, this is a good one*, I thought. She was a younger pup already socialized --- exactly what I was searching for. Having just sent my sixth boxer, Bella to the Rainbow Bridge, I figured an adolescent Number Seven could take me into later years. I had had my Number One, Angel for her full ten years. All those in-between were senior rescues: their stays with me lasting a few years only and in two cases, mere months. As their final *hooman*, my heart warmed to know that each ended their life in a loving home. Back then, the people at Boxer Rescue LA called me their Leisure World.

Cassie's stubby snout and slightly turned up nose

below a wrinkly brow and flat-top head but with natural ears exemplified classic Boxer. Only her long tail
said otherwise as it hadn't been docked short like most
Boxers. I was glad though because the tip, appearing to
have been dipped in white paint, was darling. A brindle
striped coat shone in the picture and those striking light
brown eyes were mesmerizing: indeed, it seemed I was
"caramel-eyesed."

So I swiped right.

Cassie was being fostered at the West Coast Boxer Rescue shelter headquarters in Roland Heights and
on the appointed meet-and-greet day, I faced a dreaded
freeway drive up the 60 – ugh. High speed maneuvering
is bad enough but I especially hate that two lane drag
strip where the highway passes between the mountains.
I set out, knuckles white, stopping at my usual Star-
bucks off the Chino Boulevard offramp for a pee break.
Though the shelter was only a few more miles up the
road, from there on it was bumper-to-bumper. Damn,
I was going to be late. Stuck behind a semi, a feeling of
familiarity came over me.

My mind flashed back to some twenty-plus years
earlier, before my boxer families, sitting in similar traffic.
That time I was on the 405 in Los Angeles, inching my

way on a Friday evening to dinner at a friend's house. I cursed when I took a wrong off-ramp and had to traverse side streets to get back on the freeway. *I should just turn around and go home*, I considered. But I didn't and upon arrival was led to the dining room and a table already filled with food. There, sitting among his in-laws, was a handsome, muscular man with cropped gray hair wearing a white tee shirt and blue shorts. His smile broadened as he rose his 6-foot-2 to greet me. My heart leapt. I read something special in steel blue eyes shining behind unkempt eyebrows. Although seventeen years my senior and from a wildly different background, he seemed to return the chemistry and by evening's end we both recognized our future. Meeting the man who would shortly become my husband was clearly worth four-lane torment. I realize now that the lesson learned on perseverance from that night would be one I'd practice again.

Leonid spoke little English and my command of his language, Russian was non-existent. Our first date was just the two of us plunged into a comical game of Pictionary. But we persisted with our match made in Heaven.

I was blessed with only a brief time with my precious Leonid: a time spent laughing and playing and learning how to communicate, never knowing how quickly it would all end, but intense, nonetheless. Our battle with his brain tumor came three years after that dinner. It was a fight that would introduce me first to hope then to heartbreak.

"Ya lublu tebia" is about all of his language I can remember now. It's been replaced with "What-a-baby-got." Not replaced, however, was a deadly serious pursuit of victory over cancer: a campaign I first waged those decades ago. This time, however, it would not end in heartbreak but instead in a game of catch.

PACK MENTALITY

Some years ago, I was delighted to hear Pope Francis's confirmation that "All dogs go to Heaven." It was a casual response, I suppose, to someone's query but it warmed the hearts of us Catholic pet owners, nonetheless. Recently, however, he disappointed me when he seemed to dismiss animals by stating that good Catholics must not supplant human procreation and nurturing with trans-species bonding. In essence I was being told that my canine family was a sin. In making this edict, my otherwise tolerant and broad-minded Spiritual Leader, I believe, just didn't understand. I can attest that the pet/caregiver lifestyle produces as dynamic a contribution to the Spirit of Life as can the child/parent bond, albeit in its own special way.

Partly by circumstance and somewhat by choice, I have not given birth to human children. I have, however, elected to create a pack of canines, all Boxers now totaling seven, with no regrets. One by one, my adopted kids taught me how to enjoy life unconditionally as I learned that the word 'parent' is both a noun and a verb.

11

I parented my first Boxer, Angel her entire life and tolerated her typical breed stubbornness to not 'come,' 'sit,' or 'stay.' I fed her, bathed her, and picked up her soupy poop. We enjoyed the 'walking dance' each morning and cuddled in front of the TV each night. I had her teeth cleaned and hired dog sitters to maintain her comfort at home while I traveled on business. After jumping our six-foot fence and zooming up and down our block, she taught me that all my screaming couldn't cajole her back home. Research described how humping my leg was her effort to be 'top dog' and was not to be interpreted as sexual. The mailbox on the front porch got moved when our postal carrier refused service because of her barking through the adjacent window. I dealt with Angel's food allergies, discovered the neighbors she liked and those she didn't and appreciated her preference for sleeping only at the foot of the bed.

A friend, the artist of renown Chuck Caplinger painted an incredible portrait of her in her youthful prime. I cherished how he caught

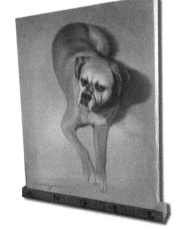

the human-like quality of her facial expression. Alas, her stubby snout slowly began its turn to gray and when the time came, I addressed her *Quality Of Life*. In my reluctant embrace with her favorite hoomans by our side, I led her to the Rainbow Bridge.

I have friends who won't adopt again because the pain of *It's time to put her down* is so heart-wrenching. We are loath to 'pull the plug' for any loved one, no matter the species, even if it is to end suffering. People intrinsically *fight on* when facing the inevitable, letting God dictate. But society has long accepted a humane option when our pets are incurable. We are allowed to make the decision to end their lives... for the good of their lives.

I'm wondering if this is the rationale behind Pope Francis' seemed change in attitude. Perhaps like his namesake, this man loves animals so much that he tacitly has removed these beings from the Church mandate that only God dictates time of death. Could this be my Papal absolution? I'd like to believe that indeed it is and that I am forgiven.

Doing nothing less for Angel than I would have done for any child from my loins, by the end of those ten years my parenting had become second nature. As I continued to grow my canine family I became inured to those inevitable sad *Goodbyes* and planted a rose bush for each memory.

From the next rescue, my water-loving Lois I learned that aggression sometimes can't be overcome and precautions must be taken. From my comical old Bubba I learned to keep a drool towel in every room. From obedient Sarge I learned that addiction to oxytocin can be stronger than life itself. From long-legged super model Heidi I learned canine "singing" need only be coaxed by the first notes of a harmonica. From Bella I learned how non-stop kisses and a sweet disposition can easily result in a foster 'fail.'

And from Cassie I learned how the spirit of a puppy, seemingly *normal* by all outward appearance but with a danger brewing inside, could persevere through an onslaught of distress that would crush the vitality of most… until the arrival of a miracle cure.

As our honeymoon months progressed, Cassie's youthful zest faded and was replaced by questions. Day by day, she would wearily get off the couch, pick up a toy and then drop back down after a few steps, toy still in mouth. So often she sniffed at her bowl only to turn away with a retch. As I sought medical diagnosis for her increasing *dis-ease*, she neither whined with complaint nor fought the probing. I never considered any of the seemingly well-meaning admonitions to put Cassie down. Something about her determination to rebound wouldn't allow even the thought that it was time to choose her rose. Enduring it all, she trusted my lead and waited with me in faithful expectation for an answer.

Maybe by instinct, maybe sheer willpower, or maybe our pack had a talk with God, once we found the solution, Cassie's promise as heir apparent became happily fulfilled.

THE PLAY'S THE THING

The Boxer breed has a well-known reputation for acting like puppies 'til the day they die. And how fun it is to play with Cassie now that she has the energy and I have the time. Emerging from the backyard heaps of stuffed squeaky toys with today's favorite in her mouth, Cassie compels me away from some project with her imploring caramel-colored eyes. Naturally, I abandon my work to wrestle Lamb Chop from her determined grip for a toss. During those few happy moments, my chore is forgotten.

I wouldn't say I had a particularly joyous childhood. My over-extended parents raised our family in Middle Of Nowhere, Missouri on an acre of softly rolling land. Arriving in the second half of our brood of seven, I was a chubby baby that grew to plump then obese, hence was the easy butt of my siblings' taunts. Their name-calling, particularly that one "*Slub*," kicked me to the bottom of the family rung and taught me my place. Though outnumbered, my butterball legs scrambled nonetheless, finding escape in a world of pretend.

Recreation in our regulated family was scarce so I treasured building forts for the kittens, watching Gilligan's Island on TV, or playing with my Barbie doll. With our Boxer, General by my side, Barbie and I would go on jungle adventures under the rhubarb plant or explore a volcano in Dad's big, rough-hewn bar-be-que. Hunting for diamonds amongst the charcoal, the mess made by General nosing through the greasy ashes was well-worth the spanking I got 'cause like my namesake, I was the pretty, skinny daredevil of my imagination.

Forty hours a week Dad designed mechanics for aerospace, then came back down to earth to build our two story, four bedroom, flat-roofed brick house all by himself. Spanning ages from not-quite teens to barely toddlers, we kids were Dad's crew drafted during the years of our youth for the property's grunt work: dumping gravel, bucket by heavy bucket, into the septic tank's deep dark hole; plowing, planting and endlessly weeding the massive vegetable garden; or holding 2x4 braces as Dad poured out cement structures. When we would complete a task and dare run off to play, Dad would gruffly call out our seven names in age-descending order and reprimand, "You're not excused! Ask for another job before you leave." I'd lower my eyes and ask dutifully, cringing, because there always was another chore. So, the TV remained black, Barbie stayed in her box, and General slept on a blanket for another day.

As we grew, Mom went back to nursing. One hazy memory is of her giving polio vaccines to a long line of uniformed kids at our school. Somehow, she'd fit in working outside the house alongside family duties and running the community 4-H club. Under her leadership, we learned to cook and sew. Stylish in her 50's fashions and well-documented in Dad's home movies, Mom kept six daughters and herself clothed. She even made her own hats. We four older girls shared the household chores and babysat the two toddlers: always keeping busy with little time to play.

I had to pull double duty helping Dad. When our only brother, the oldest, Mark went off to college I was drafted as the substitute boy of the family. A layer of fat insulated me from cold winter hours spent holding the flashlight while Dad changed a fuse or rebuilt a carburetor. Hearing my sisters' merriment upstairs, I fumed that I was stuck indentured. Though totally unfair, utterly boring and seldom receiving any praise for the help, these stints satisfied a craving my childhood brain didn't realize: rare alone-time with a parent. I laughed at his dumb jokes, rolled my eyes at his stern advice ("You need to develop a thick skin, Hon,") and always asked for another job when the task was finished. Memory doesn't serve when he started calling me "Hon." Shortened from "Honey," it became his precious - and life-long – nickname for me.

As their nest began to empty the folks relocated us to California where I truly came into my own. A ten-cent bus ride provided temporary escape from Dad's renovations: time in the sun exploring the offerings of a big city with school friends who didn't call me mean names. Perhaps recognizing something I didn't, Mom signed me up for drama class in school. She worked nursing during the swing shift at a beach-front hospital and when I got my driver's license, we shared Gram's clunky Nash Rambler for commutes to and from my evening play rehearsals and her job. Once home each night, we'd decompress together at the kitchen table before going to bed.

Over a cup of tea or bowl of ice cream (sometimes with an alcoholic douse of crème de menthe) she'd hear all about the school's latest production and my amateur attempts at method acting. I'd ask about her patients and the staff on the ward. Her stories of nursing during WWII were fascinating. Our chats were no longer mother-daughter: we talked like roommates. Then she made an easy pivot back to motherhood sewing all my costumes for the plays.

When British elegance was needed for my senior turn in an Oscar Wilde opus, she found thrift store draperies of ornate brocade for the fabric and we laughed together at this very *Scarlet O'Hara* solution. Throughout the coming years, Mom tailored all my finest couture. In her loving creations' embrace I walked down the aisle and up the red carpet.

By its very definition, a career in the entertainment industry could fulfill my long-starved appetite to pretend. Enjoying every demanding but glorious minute, my profession sent me on adventures that no soot-covered little girl could ever imagine.

It's said that good luck happens when opportunity meets preparedness. I'm not exactly sure when I recognized that Dad's dreaded childhood chores guided my work ethic and Mom's crafty ingenuity contributed to my accolades. I just know that I relish their example set.

During the years before they passed, I'd often phone 'Our Nurse,' Mom seeking medical advice for some malady or share plans with Dad on a backyard project. My monthly weekend visits before their slow ascent to Heaven found us playing dominos or tackling crosswords puzzles. "You have such good printing, Hon," Dad once told me. "You would have made a good engineer."

After Sunday Mass, we might go to the dog park for zoomies. Watching my Boxer at play would send Dad's memory back to General running around the old brick house. Mom smiled at his reverie, enjoying the warmth of the sun. We'd eat dessert watching a black and white film on Turner Classic Movies. Afterwards, my pup and I would be sent on our way home with "When are you coming back, Hon?"

Full circle, we three embraced our inner child together having finally found the time to play.

NOT FOR THE SQUEAMISH

"Out, out damn-ed spot!" says mad Lady Mac-Beth... or rather in my mind, says Katherine Hepburn, her distinctive accent delivering the line from a favorite movie. Repeating this mantra keeps me hands-and-knees-motivated scrubbing kitchen tile grout lines blackened by drippings of Cassie's bodily fluids. My body aches on the hard porcelain and my fingers are raw, encrusted with the baking soda/hydrogen peroxide formula I concocted for the job (*but hey, it works.*) Only the far corners have missed discoloration from nearly three years of constant wiping up of doggy vaginal discharge but I'm determined to accomplish my New Year's resolution to *finally* deep clean the entire house now that the likelihood of further staining is past.

And indeed, Cassie's plight approached the Shakespearean. Beginning only a few months after adopting each other, on a day in May 2018 I saw a moist spot on the floor after Cassie stood up from a sit. A trip to the vet brought diagnosis as a common urinary tract infection. This discharge progressed over that summer as those mere spots became puddles, concerning me more and more that something was really wrong with my recent rescue. She had joined me here at her *fur-ever* home just that spring in supposed perfect health. Our *getting-to-know-you* had barely started.

"Sometimes rescue dogs have underlying issues," our vet, Dr. Rachel Reedy suggested. Calmly professional yet baby-faced, dark-haired Dr. Reedy had been my vet of choice for several years. She compassionately cared for Cassie's pack-sister, Bella with her lymphoma, relieving her pain and ultimately helping me send her to the Rainbow Bridge. I trusted Dr. Reedy's knowledge with my new little pocket Boxer but many questions about Cassie went unanswered, "Maybe she's still adjusting to her new life?" So Dr. Reedy wrote us another script for antibiotics to stop the odd liquid dripping from her vagina.

It didn't stop and by July, Cassie had become a regular at the vet's office where the staff fawned over her generous kisses during every visit. Yet more examinations and blood tests showed nothing to explain the dripping from her vaginal area, so back on Amoxicillin Cassie went. The antibiotic was at least a temporary stop to the symptom.

"It works and it can't hurt," Dr. Reddy said.

One day in early August my alarm heightened. I noticed that the area from under Cassie's tail down to her "privates" seemed puffy – swollen maybe. Then I saw that the ubiquitous fluid on the floor sometimes had a slight pink tinge. *Okay, this is definitely not normal,* I thought, growing frantic to find out what the heck was wrong with my little girl.

I am no prude. Over the course of my past six Boxers, I've cleaned my share of yellow bile vomit and explosive soupy poops. They call it "Boxer colitis" for a reason and I knew what I was in for after parenting so many of this breed. Although I had never adopted a puppy thus experienced a dog going through heat, I knew this couldn't possibly be the cause of Cassie's drips: I had a copy of her spay certificate.

I reached out to West Coast Boxer Rescue from which I adopted Cassie and spoke with Jackie, my point person there. She confirmed that I was told the exact same information that they were given by the lady, one of their regular rescuers, who delivered Cassie to them. Jackie offered the woman's phone number which I used.

"I'm desperate to find out what's wrong with Cassie. Do you know *any* of her medical history?" I begged in my phone call to this woman. With a distinct Italian accent, she began a litany of what I had already been told: Cassie was rescued from a backyard breeder situation in Chula Vista where it was overcrowded; Cassie was pure bred (the woman said she saw the Boxer bitch and sire personally;) the breeders were purposely mating for the more popular smaller-sized Boxers; and she was spayed in Tijuana, a usual practice in the San Diego area because it was cheaper there. *Okay, this all seems logical.*

She told me that Cassie had had mange, probably from the over-crowded conditions at the breeders. *That was news to me.* And then she said that the Mexican vet *admitted* that he performed a partial spay.

"Wait, what?" I asked. "What's a 'partial' spay?" Talking rapidly, she tried to explain full vs. partial spay logistics but I couldn't discern from her confusing words if Cassie's uterus or ovaries had been removed by the Tijuana vet. This was not making a hell of a lot of sense and her rather cavalier attitude with these revelations raised the hairs on my neck. "And what do you mean he '*admitted*' the partial spay?" By now I was jotting down everything she said.

I shared this newly learned history with Dr.

Reedy who supposed that the deep wrinkles on Cassie's face were actually scars from the mange (*one question answered.*) She told me that sometimes vets in third world countries remove just the dog's uterus and leave the ovaries: basically, sterilization via hysterectomy. She ordered a progesterone hormone test, which proved "inconclusive."

I Googled all this educating myself on canine reproductive systems. By now Cassie's vaginal drips had progressed to a brighter pink. My internet search bar filled with every condition's keyword of which I could think and I printed out the resulting possible diseases no matter how remote. Though aware that most medical professionals dearly hate internet diagnoses, I didn't care 'cause we had no answers otherwise.

Growing tired of scrubbing upholstery (I should have bought stock in Oxyclean,) I covered all the furniture in the house with towels which required daily changing. With relief, antibiotics would stop Cassie's dripping for a week or so... then to my dismay, it would resume. Some months later I'd discover the joys of doggy diapers but during those early days I kept tissues in every pocket for mop up and cringed when she went into one of those full body adjustment shakes, spewing red splatters everywhere. The bleeding really didn't seem to bother Cassie, although I was amazed at her contortions when cleaning herself *down there*.

A playful, barely three-year old puppy, she was devoted to the piles of stuffed squeaky toys she inherited from my previous Boxers, our pack of six watching over us from the Rainbow Bridge. We'd play catch in the backyard atop the concrete patio now mottled with her red drops baking in the summer sun. I sort of liked the design created on the boring gray deck, growing increasingly gory as any TV crime scene could be staged. I stuttered to think what luminol might display throughout my property. My fruitless lunges to catch a droplet off the tip of her vulva were surely comical.

As mystified as I was, rescue lady Jackie set up a phone consultation with Dr. Clark, Chief of Staff at Western University Veterinarian College, who suggested a second spay which Dr. Reedy dutifully performed. Once again, *inconclusive*.

"Her uterus was atrophied," the good doctor reported after the operation, "...just a stump. Maybe the first spay removed the uterus and left the ovaries? I found no infection, no accumulated blood, everything looks normal in that area." We were still in the dark.

Cassie recovered from the unnecessary procedure with her usual indomitable spirit, and alas the bleeding resumed thicker, now burgundy colored. The conundrum that this mysterious and utterly gross affliction was happening to an otherwise healthy dog was not lost on any of us. Dr. Reedy surmised that the current clot-dotted discharge could be a hold-over from the operation and prescribed more Amoxicillin, which had become the one and only effective bleeding abatement, albeit temporarily.

"Otherwise," she said, "I just have no idea."

In early December, our Amoxicillin supply had run out. I called Dr. Reedy's office to refill the 'script but got voicemail. I didn't receive a return call that day and Cassie's bleeding was a steady flow again. Local TV evening news reported that the owner of a veterinarian office, *my* veterinarian office, was involved in some kind of scandal and had locked its doors leaving Dr. Reedy and staff facing a 'closed' sign on the front door and un-informed patients behind them in the parking lot with no re-opening date. Desperate for a new drug dealer, I was relieved to get an appointment with another local vet.

As Cassie and I waited in the exam room at Paws

and Claws Urgent Care in nearby Palm Desert on that chilly morning, my anxiety was at an all-time high. I've always had white-coat syndrome… plus I had a very convoluted story to tell… and Cassie dripping red blops all over the floor didn't help. Bent over to wipe up the blood, my butt greeted the person who came through the door.

"Sorry about that," I said, dropping the red-tinged tissues in the waste can.

Tall and athletic with a shock of curly grayish hair and wearing requisite monotone scrubs, Dr. Alexis Rambaud replied easily, "No problem," as she lowered herself to Cassie's level. She asked me what was going on. I pulled out a bound, monthly calendar on which I had been keeping daily track of Cassie's symptoms. Tucked inside were all my Googled research printouts. As I recounted Cassie's symptoms and speculative causes gleaned from the internet, Dr. Rambaud ran her hands gently over Cassie's body. I noticed henna-style tattoos on her hands and more tats running up her arms from behind the long sleeves. There was something about that ink that distracted my apprehension.

Dr. Rambaud listened to my recitation as she softly pressed on that swollen area above Cassie's privates. I was relieved that she gave credence to my account since that closed, scandal-ridden vet office couldn't supply Cassie's files. Not unexpectedly, she ordered the usual tests and suggested an ultrasound. Accommodating my request, the doctor had a script for Amoxicillin called in to our CVS.

Rubbing behind Cassie's ears, she then surprised me with the question, "Would you consider a holistic approach?" She looked into Cassie's caramel eyes and asked her, "Would you like that?" Dr. Rambaud handed me a small green and white box covered in Chinese printing. "Let's try this too. It's called Yunnan Baiyao… Chinese soldiers used it in combat to stop bleeding. It works." Once home I Googled it. Cassie soon proved them all right: the bleeding stopped.

This new hope in hand would become a first life-vest in Cassie's upcoming three-year voyage through a sea of troubles, and Dr. Rambaud signed on as our Captain to end them.

A BITCH OF A DAY

I'm not one to call people names. I've been called too many of 'em throughout my days as "*Fatty Fatty Two By Four*" that I try not to, normally, inflict verbal insults upon someone else. But I've made a *grand exception* for The Lying Bitch, an exception which in my opinion is well deserved. Let me be clear: because of my decades' long tenure as a dog parent, the term 'bitch' holds a neutral connotation, that of being a 'female dog,' which I use in everyday conversation. But in this one case, I willfully inflict upon this specific moniker every contrary and adverse meaning I can possibly sling in her direction, starting from that busy mid-January day.

Barely finishing my grandé before getting the call from Desert Veterinary Specialists to come pick up Cassie, I had anticipated a much longer wait for the ultrasound test to be completed. Only ninety minutes before, Cassie and I arrived for her appointment early as is my usual habit. I always give myself a little extra time when I'm driving someplace new and the morning drizzle prompted our departure from home even more so.

Cassie didn't mind. She loved car rides, jumping up and down in anticipation as I tussled to get her harness over her head and under her front limbs. Before allowing her to vault into the Toyota's back seat, I checked to make sure the pink blanket covered it entirely, tucking in the corners and around the padded center hump stool just to make sure. A blood-stained blanket can be washed but permanent damage to the upholstery was something I preferred to avoid. *Maybe I should double up,* I thought in anticipation of a long ride, struggling to secure her harness to the seat belt. Cassie used the opportunity to sneak in a quick face lick.

I didn't need that extra time to get to our destination. The parking lot in front of the nondescript vet building was empty. Dodging droplets, we had a few minutes to kill before they opened and I wondered if she sensed that I was nervous about the test results. Cassie had no idea what would be happening to her today. She was interested only in the critter odors on the curb. Hoping she'd have one good pee before the procedure, I braved the rain and she squatted. "Good girl. Good *outside*," I told her, reinforcing my dog-speak command for "pee" as her stream covered some other dog's scent. Smiling from behind the glass front door, a petite woman unlocked it to start the day and motioned at us to come out of the rain. Cassie affably greeted the young lady as we entered. Within minutes, they were *best buds*.

The clouds had parted while I waited at a Bucky's down the street. I barely had started the crossword from a discarded newspaper when my Samsung rang. "Wow, that was fast," I said to Cassie's new buddy on the phone.

The young lady told me that Cassie had been perfectly calm and thus no sedative was required for the ultrasound so I could come pick her up. She said that Dr. Allett would like to discuss the results with me.

In the bright consultation room, Cassie pawed at Dr. Allett playfully wanting his attention. "The ultrasound shows nothing out of the ordinary," he reported. I let out a breath of relief then familiar concern crept back in. "I didn't see any masses and her organs are all of normal size," he said as his finger circled over the gray monochrome film showing Cassie's insides backlit on an LED screen. He explained a logistical problem, however: the probe doesn't 'read' past Cassie's pelvic bones so that area (the area of our concern) could not be included in the scan. He showed me the section on Cassie's behind where those opaque bones were, petting along her back as he did so.

Oh, Good Lord, why did I even do this expensive test in the first place? I thought, immediately answering the question to myself. I knew full well the importance of ruling things *out*. I reminded Dr. Allett of the 'partial spay' advice we had been told and he confirmed to my surprise that he saw no evidence of Cassie's ovaries: they must have indeed been removed in the original spay.

"How could that be?" I wondered out loud.

He shook his head, "They're not there." Answering the proverbial chicken-or-egg question (she no longer had either uterus or ovaries,) the puzzle as to the source of the bleeding remained. I asked what he would do going forward were Cassie his dog. "The only option now is exploratory surgery," he recommended, fondling behind her ears. He promised to call our referring vet, Dr. Rambaud with the results and then asked that I keep him informed of what we find out. "Cassie's a sweetheart," he said more to her than to me. "She's got such beautiful eyes."

Riding shotgun from the backseat going home, Cassie stood on the center divider and gave me wet willies with her tongue as she is wont to do all the while entranced by the boulevard scenery ahead. She seemed none the worse for wear and I relished her affection, happy at how well she had cooperated with the prob-ing. "I heard you were a good girl," I proudly told her, reaching back to cup her jowls and wipe the slobber off my neck. As she settled down for the ride, the question marks from the morning test results popped back into my brain. By the time we arrived home, my determina-tion to find answers was renewed. I must go back to the beginning.

Searching the phone's September call log histo-ry, my fingers shook though I'm not really sure why. I pressed redial and recognized the Italian accented voice that answered. Perhaps this lady, the one who had de-livered Cassie to the rescue people and later told of the now questionable '*admitted*' partial spay, heard that the tone of my voice was different from when we had talked before. I quickly recounted the past months of Cassie's increasing bloody discharge, the frustrating lack of diagnosis, all the antibiotics and Yunnan Baiyao, plus that morning's ultrasound that disproved her advice of a 'fix' procedure that may have been out of the ordinary.

Summoning all my resolve, I implored for more details about that Tijuana spay operation. I needed to speak with that vet. "Would you please help me get ahold of him?" I begged.

I asked her about the backyard breeders. I needed to know if her condition might be congenital and if Cassie had possibly bled from birth. "Can I contact them?" I asked, growing more demanding.

She responded telling me that Cassie wasn't in Chula Vista until *after* she was in Tijuana. I pulled out the paper on which I had jotted notes from our first conversation.

"That's not what you told me in September," I countered. "You said she came from a backyard breeder in Chula Vista... that she was taken to the Tijuana vet for her spay 'cause it was cheaper there than in the States."

She answered no: Cassie was found on the streets of Tijuana, *then* she went to Chula Vista. She added that Cassie had mange.

Addressing the second thing she just said, I replied, "You told me that in September."

Then she said that Cassie had had TVT.

I went silent, and asked her to say that again.

She repeated that Cassie had TVT.

"What does that stand for?" I asked and wrote

down 'T' 'V' 'T' on that same piece of paper.

She rattled off long words. Transmisa... mumble... mumble... tumor... What she said was undiscernible and sounded meaningless to me. Then she quickly added that Cassie was cured. One hundred percent. She was cured, she assured me... *before* she was sent to the States for adoption.

"So Cassie didn't come from a backyard breeder?" I asked. I wasn't understanding. "You didn't really meet Cassie's parents?"

The rest of the conversation was a blur: the woman's voice became unintelligible with increasingly heavy Italian cadence; jumbling timelines and explanations; in a hurry to get off the phone. That was the last time I spoke with this woman. Then and forever she would be known to me as The Lying Bitch.

Trying to process this new revelation, I stood immobilized in my home office while Cassie nudged my leg, toy in mouth for play. Booting up my desktop, I tossed her toy to chase and phoned Dr. Rambaud, leaving a message for her to call me as soon as possible.

Canine *Transmissible Venereal Tumor.* A Googled medical study outlined the basics: benign genital reticuloendothelial (*I must Google this word*) lesion common in third world countries with uncontrolled canine populations; etiology (*Google this word*) by cell transplant from affected to unaffected dogs; manifesting in the subcutaneous (*Google this word*) tissue which bleeds and ulcerates; frequently deforming the perineal (*Google this word*) region; antigenic (*Google this word*) and highly effected by the host's immune response during the progressive and regressive (*Google this word*) stages; a considerable hemorrhagic (*Google this word*) vulvar discharge may occur; can either metastasize or regress spontaneously after logarithmic (*Google this word*) growth; is known to recur in ten percent of treated cases often becoming chemo-resistant where the cure rate is lower.

I wondered why this hadn't popped up in any of my prior Googled searches. Maybe my layman nomenclature was to blame. With so many new questions I implored in my head, *Please, Dr. Rambaud. Please, call me back*, and read on. The Treatment section of the study contained even longer, more foreign sounding medical words, blurry on the screen from the tears that filled my eyes.

Why, in God's name, didn't The Lying Bitch tell me about Cassie's so very serious disease in our first conversation? Why did she make up stories about *back-yard breeders*? What was all that *I saw her parents myself* bullshit? Couldn't that Bitch have told me the truth in the first place about how this innocent puppy, a *perra callejera* street dog, was raped by a dog whose infected penis had injected her with a cancer?

September, October, November, December and now January: months of time lost to only questions and no proactive treatment to stem the disease. Time wasted allowing the tumor in Cassie to selfishly grow; empowering it against the upcoming onslaught of chemotherapies; granting it strength to overcome any antidote; all possibly beyond hope.

How could a person, supposedly devoted to rescue, purposely do this to a dog?

To such a precious dog?

To my Cassie?

FINDING CIARA

I admit it. I'm hooked. Daily – okay more than just daily – I jones for my fix. As deft as a teenager, I grasp my addiction: scrolling through posts and memes; whirling past ads and alternative facts; *liking* and *hearting* with a dexterity that belies my arthritis. The social media endorphin rush that is Facebook, with all its publicized faults, connects me to *The World*, but it's not really the world. Rather, it's an insular *metaverse* that exists only on the internet.

Cassie hates my enslavement of course. The moment I pick up the glowing rectangle that is my smartphone, all hopes of a romp with her Hooman are dashed. Yes, I feel guilty, but little does she know what an important tool Facebook was with her mystery.

More powerful than this obsession, however, was my determination to find details that the second phone call with the Italian liar didn't provide. On that Bitch of an Afternoon, I reported to Dr. Rambaud about the perplexing revelation imparted by she-whose-real-name-shall-never-again-cross-my-lips. Other than the diagnosis, I could share nothing definitive about treatment, dosage or dates: only advice from a woman who, as far as I could tell, lied about everything else.

"What do we do now?" I asked the vet.

"An exploratory vaginoscopy is the only way to know for sure. If we find a mass, we'll do a biopsy," she said. Just that morning the ultrasound vet had recommended this as well. Dr. Rambaud promised staff would call back with the cost. Her voice seemed skeptical about the diagnosis, "TVT treatments are usually successful. If Cassie was treated as you were told, the tumor should not have come back. However, this disease is rare in the States… I've never treated a case of TVT even once. I'll do some research." I offered to share the Googled studies I found about TVT. "Let's not assume anything until we get the biopsy results."

The vaginoscopy was scheduled for the following week.

Facing seven days of worry, I turned back to my desktop. TVT search results displayed scientific theses by veterinarians in Thailand, Greece, India, Viet Nam, another from Greece, Argentina, and more from Thailand. Every one of them described how an infected male dog 'implants' the contagious tumor in the female dog during intercourse. The accompanying pictures of fleshy pink cauliflower-like bumps on dog penises turned my stomach and the bulbous backsides of females' internal growths angered my imagination. Each paper cited Cassie's symptoms to a tee and all prescribed six weeks of vincristine sulfate as the *go-to* chemotherapy cure. *Was this the "cure" that Cassie got?* I assumed so...

Googling unrecognizable medical words along the way, I was becoming an expert. The papers stated that the cancer, also known as *Sticker's sarcoma,* can possibly metastasize to other parts of the body, but that's rare. *There's a relief,* I thought. One important differentiation I learned was that unlike the usual cause of cancer - a bodily-cell dysfunction for instance - this unique tumor is spread by *implantation.* Cassie's body was perfectly healthy *sans tumor.* The cancer was *put upon* her earning its name "Transmissible."

Then I found something more immediately alarming.

Alongside the studies' pictures of defiled canine genitals were some depicting nasty-looking nasal lesions. Excuse me: *tumors in their noses?* Short of kinky doggy sex, how would the tumor cells get up the nose?

45

Holy crap, I thought, *through sniffing! Common everyday Spot-meet-Fido/Fido-meet-Spot backside sniffing!* My mind flashed immediately to the last time I picked Cassie up from doggy day care.

CONTAGEOUS! OMG! My Cassie could have been spreading a malignant contagion at day care! I made a quick phone call to my East Coast-based lawyer, Alex Murphy. Luckily, I caught him before he had ended his day. I told him of Cassie's predicament and with trembling voice, read to him the day care facility directive I had signed averring that Cassie was healthy with no communicable disease. *Am I liable if another dog caught TVT from Cassie's mucus-y backside? Might there be a playmate of Cassie's harboring the disease in its nostrils?* With a reassuring confidence, he deftly recited legalities covering negligence and liability then offered that I did not *knowingly* expose the canine populace, nor could I have known about the disease given our bona fide circumstances and the fact that I'm not a veterinarian.

"So, I'm not liable," I said letting out the breath I had been holding. "Besides," I assured myself aloud, "We won't know for sure if Cassie has TVT until the biopsy." He insisted that even if she's positive, I had no legal exposure. Thank God… and thank you, Alex. I needed a break from Google so I opened a different tab in Firefox to indulge my Facebook habit.

There's nothing more delightful than scrolling through pictures of lovable Boxers. After too many years of mind-deluding crap that sapped the sanity of nearly half of America, Facebook owns its share of our political mess, but its proliferation of pet pictures earns the app my continued usage. Long ago I recognized all the propaganda garbage and used *delete post* habitually. I prefer its by-invitation-only groups: private sets of known and trusted cadres of *friends*. My favorite is called "Once A Boxer Lover, Always A Boxer Lover," which then changed its name to "Furringdomland" to include pets of all breeds and species. Started by some Boxer-loving ladies in Greece, our animal-loving group hoomans now number over 800 and spans nearly every nation.

I first 👍*ed* the page back when I had Bella, my Number Six. I'd share pictures to the group-feed of Bella cuddling her stuffies or dressed in our Mrs. Claus Christmas costume. The members offered advice about the weird bump on her paw and shared recipes for homemade treats. My posted pix and videos garnered 🤍*s* from all over the world and I, in turn, 🤍*ed* their adorable pets too. These on-line *friends-I've-never-met* shared pain relief suggestions when Bella's lymphoma was diagnosed and they 😢*ed* with me when she made her voyage to the Bridge.

Furringdomland had become my pack. As close as any blood relations, my click of a button, *family-by-choice* support group inherently suffers no long-wrought issues to avoid. The Athens-based administrators were Nicha and her cutie-patootie boy, Idefix plus Vivi with her beauty, Athena. There were many, many more: Diane and the adorable Zena who lived in Canada; Melanie and little Theo in the UK; Cris and her darling mix-breed dubbed 'Froggie' in Sao Paolo; and the super-rescuer who never turned down a dog in need, Juno who, with her pack of five were in Houston. I could go on and on and on naming all my fellow hooman *FB* friends….

Through their posts, I came to know our group members and their pets of course and naturally they were all delighted when I adopted Cassie. Mystified alongside me about her odd symptoms, they offered various possibilities for diagnosis (some fairly screwy, some of serious consideration) in those early months. Escape to their on-line comradery would distract my worry that day. I posted to my Facebook family the frustrations about being in the dark on Cassie's (*unknown?*) treatment by the Tijuana vet. I desperately needed information on what was happening to her and appreciated the ability to vent, albeit virtually. One member, I don't remember who but it could have been any of them, asked, "Does the vet in Tijuana have a Facebook page?" *Ooooh, there's a thought…*

In the *search* bar I typed the name of the vet from Cassie's spay certificate. Click. There it was! I started scrolling through the Spanish language posts and clicked on some of the dogs pictured at the facility: most were emaciated; some wore plaster casts; others laid languid on blankets. Though I didn't understand the Spanish language comments, the photos broke my heart. *Could there be a photo of Cassie?* I wondered, and went to retrieve Cassie's original spay certificate. Calculating how far back I would need to scroll to reach her spay date, I squinted to discern from the bad photocopy the 'name' entry which had been crossed out and replaced with "*Cassie.*" I began my search again for her original name: "Ciara."

Scroll.

Scroll.

Scroll.

Scroll.

Scroll.

Finally reaching early 2017, I found no posting for a "Ciara." *Damn.* I noticed a name that popped up more than just frequently in the vet's *comment* sections: Nancy Goodwin. This name was all over the feed. *I wonder who she is?*

It was time for dinner so I abandoned my desktop pursuit. Cassie headed out the back door for a pee, dripping pink along the way including *splat*, a big one right on the threshold rug. I sighed with a pained grunt, *It's so much easier to clean blood off the tiles, Cassie. Maybe work on your aim...?*

Once we were both sated, Cassie snuggled on her favorite chair for a post-meal nap and I grabbed my smartphone to continue the mission, but not before tucking another drip towel under Cassie's backside. Settled on the sofa, I turned on the television for some white noise and multi-tasking. Switching devices meant I had to start my scrolling activity from the beginning. Digestion sapped my brain energy making another fruitless scroll through the vet's Facebook page *no bueno.*

Instead, I clicked on the Nancy Goodwin name and scrolled anew. So many sad dog photos paged by. With wanton voyeurism, I marveled at her unabashed solicitations to Facebook friends asking for donations on behalf of these dogs in need. Surgeries, medicines, chemotherapy, transport and more all required funding. Scrolling backward in time - week by week - month by month – this Nancy Goodwin lady was some kind of doggy guardian angel… and boy did she know a lot of rich people! The donations rolled in: fifty dollars here; a hundred dollars there.... It was amazing how many *perros callejeros* were getting treatment from just this one woman's Facebook advocacy even though her 'about' page said she's located in Belgium. God Bless her.

Scroll.

Scroll.

Scroll.

Scroll.

Scroll.

Then I found it. I sat upright so quickly that Cassie stirred in her slumber. It was a before-and-after photo montage of a dog, gray mange incrusted, in the upper left corner progressing to a brindle-coated puppy smiling for the camera in the lower right. A heart shaped kite flew over the words "Ciara's Journey" in happy pink letters. Though it said "Ciara," I recognized the dog immediately. This was Cassie. Unmistakably, she was my Cassie. The post was dated February 4, 2017.

I started to weep.

I found Ciara.

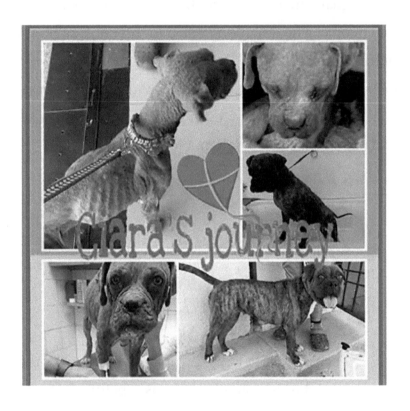

SOLILOQUY

I felt this way before… back when I was just a puppy… those funny feelings inside. The hurt back by my tail was very bad. I only wanted to sleep then. I had no hurt when I slept and I liked my dreams of chasing bunnies through the alley.

I was very happy to be with my hooman jefa *back then. She gave me food and I liked her other dogs too. Even though they looked hungry, some of them ate their food then spit it back to the dirt. Every time she gave me food the hooman made the "sssss" sound… like the snakes who'd warn me to stay away. I liked when she gently touched me where it didn't hurt. I would hear her make the snake sound "*sscciara*" so I ran to her for some-thing good, even though it hurt to run. I looked in her eyes and I heard "*Ciara.*" That was my special word. I learned other words too. And I learned that this hooman was good.*

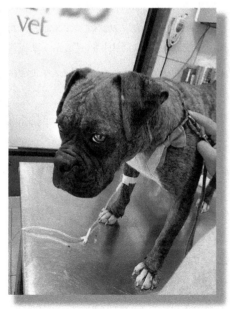

She walked me to a white house with many small rooms and gentle hooman hands but very strange smells like I had never smelled

before.

My fur hurt all the time and the wind would burn when I ran. I liked the water the hooman hands flowed on me - it made my skin feel nice! Soon my coat didn't crack anymore and then it stopped hurting. They put a sting in my leg. After that when I ate, sometimes my food would come up from my tummy too.

The other dogs and me had many sleeps with the lady hooman, with many bowls of food that sometimes went on the dirt, and many walks to the white building. I heard sweet, song noises from the hoomans when I was a good girl (and sometimes growly ones when I was naughty.) I wanted to be a good girl for the hoomans, because they helped me feel like a puppy chasing bunnies again.

I went on a long ride with fast wind out the window, a lot of new sounds and curious smells with a hooman I didn't know. This hooman didn't make the snake sound when she gave me food. Now I heard the "kkkk" sound like when something is in my throat. I learned my new special sound was "KKKCassie" and always went where I heard it.

This hooman gave me to new hoomans who put me in my own little house with my own banket. One day I got some wonderful water again that smelled special like flowers. They put a new band around my neck and led me out of my kennel and into an open room. That was the day I jumped into some new arms... the arms of My Hooman. She made the "Cassie" sound for me. So with My Hooman we went to our fur-ever home. I could smell her everywhere. Soon my smell was everywhere too.

My skin stayed soft and the wind never hurt when My

Hooman and me played in the sun.

But after many sleeps, I could feel my inside hurt… back by my tail… again. I hoped with each sleep it would go away but the funny tasting goo dripped more and more. I licked it clean but more dripped out. My Hooman gave me many loving kisses which made my heart happy… but the hurt down there grew bigger.

She took me to a different white house with different small rooms but with gently familiar hooman hands. Like before, they put stings in my leg and My Hooman put those funny tasting things down my throat. I stayed quiet and swallowed them and I was not naughty because I hoped it will make me feel like a puppy… just like it did before.

Even if it takes many many sleeps and many many small rooms, I will be a good girl and let My Hooman bring back my happy.

QUE LINDA

"I'm so *confused!!!*" I lamented with hands either side of my head channeling my best Vinnie Barbarino in a lame attempt to lighten my mood. Confusion was understandable at this point but somewhat self-wrought. I could have just calmed down and waited for next week's scope surgery which will explore Cassie's insides. If anything is found in there, the doctor will take a piece and get a definitive, scientific result. Why was I driving myself crazy?

But Cassie was bleeding again – on and off – real red blood with each drip. I recorded the discharge on that day's square in my Boxer Rescue LA calendar beneath the montage of cute doggy faces on the facing page. Starting months prior, each square had become a hand-written diary to share with the vets. I thought it important they knew what was happening to Cassie during the times they didn't see her. Or perhaps I wanted to prove that I was telling the truth and not in the grip of *Munchausen Syndrome by Proxy.*

My Mom had been my first call on medical issues my entire life whether I was ailing, had sprained an ankle, was depressed, or suffered from a toothache. I tapped her nursing background and sought her advice which quite often might override my self-diagnosis and even that of doctors *practicing* medicine. Naturally, I called her about Cassie's first symptoms. Thus, from our daily phone conversations, Mom had been living my dog's dilemma right along with me... to the extent that she could. In these, her last years especially since Dad passed, despite blessedly decent mental cognizance, her attention was becoming more and more strained. Although she would ask *How's Cassie?* during every call, alas, confusions about my dog became taxing to my then 100 year-old Mom, so I deferred to her limitations. I stuck to inquiring about her own ailments and refrained from asking her what *antineoplastic* meant or what a *bisphosphonate* does as I might have in the past. All else was happy talk.

Neither did I seek solace from others in my life as I didn't welcome a repeat of early-on suggestions to euthanize my girl. They could not understand that other than whatever was causing the bleeding, Cassie was a healthy, normal, loving dog. I was saddened that empathy was not so strong with this group. Cassie deserved more than mere expediency.

I am blessed to have had one person, however, who truly filled the role of a supportive sister: I had Linda's shoulders to cry on. Before I moved to the desert, lovely Linda Jorgensen was my neighbor with whom I shared the Los Angeles enclave on the quiet side of LAX that is Westchester. She lived just beyond walking distance from my old house and worked at the university only a few blocks past that. We had met through a mutual friend who also worked at the college; a friend who learned of Linda's love for animals and recognized that she and I had a lot in common. Of sturdy build and with a head of thick wavy brown hair that belied the stereotypical-blond Norwegian that she was, Linda had boundless energy. Whether advocating for the college students put in her trust during her workday or spending every other waking minute of her forty-something years devoted to animals, Linda was the one who helped me sort things out from Cassie's very first anomaly.

Between weekend gigs house-sitting friends' dogs, cats, horses, even a turtle or two; working with pigeon and possum (yes, possum) rescue; and her own impressive home pack of always four or more critters, Linda couldn't turn down any opportunity for as-

59

sistance. In addition to being the beloved aunt to my Boxers throughout the years, Linda and her menageries went beyond the norm – *well* beyond the norm. Ripley, a pittie was her life-long *heart-dog.* After an admirable life as leader of the pack, in his later years Ripley fell victim to melanoma of which Linda stopped at nothing to mitigate - adding years to his time with her. Her investment in medical care and emotional heartbreak resulted in an endowment she matched financially, which kept her constantly broke.

I'm embarrassed to say that I can't keep straight all the ailments for which Linda treated her two smallest dogs, first Peanut and then Bing, nor do I remember the name of her burly pet snake. During visits I kept a safe distance from both it and its meals of mice stored in the freezer. When the snake died, he joined his dinners on ice, waiting for an appropriate memorial service, I suppose.

Linda collects old blankets for animal shelters, rents her garage studio apartment to her ex-boyfriend, home cooks food for her four-legged pack and with me had been learning all about transmissible venereal tumors. Though 100 miles divide us, Lady Linda, who defines the word *rescue,* helped me tackle my pique of confusion, spending hours on the phone sorting through Cassie's predicament. We were *Cagney and Lacey* but on Animal Planet. She was mystified along with me how, despite the aberrations, Cassie was so very 'normal.'

My phone's wake-up alarm rang early the morning of the scheduled vaginoscopy. I gave myself only a short amount of time to get dressed and out the door so that Cassie, maybe, wouldn't notice that she wasn't getting any breakfast. Our pop-culture driven world was by now well versed on propofol and veterinarian science dictates it should never be mixed with a full stomach on the operating table. No matter. After a quick elimination walk, Cassie gleefully bounded into the back seat of the car, forgetting all about food and happy to be going on a ride with her hooman.

At the vet office, I kissed her *Good-bye* and stopped on my way home for a croissant at my favorite French bakery where I texted Linda to ask when we could chat: I needed a diversion from the day's worry. Luckily, it was student conference week and she had a couple spare hours at noon.

While Cassie was ticking yet another notch on her growing list of medical procedures, Linda joined me on the phone as I put pen to paper organizing symptoms and conditions - facts and lies - past and present - what I knew and what I didn't know. We tried to sort out what swirled in my head. The list resembled a glossary for Merck's Veterinarian Manual.

With her help, I had pages and pages awaiting Dr. Rambaud's consultation. However, despite the astute organization, my mind remained a jumble.

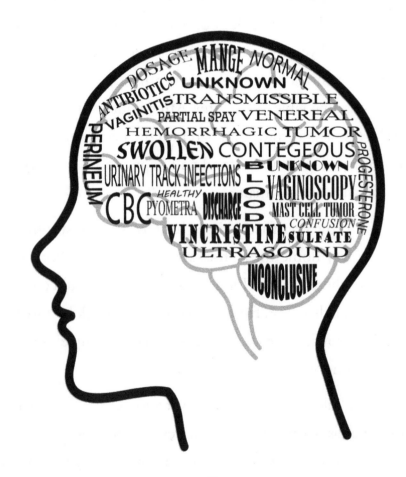

We were interrupted by an incoming call from Paws and Claws so I thanked Linda *Good-bye*. I was told Cassie was awake but groggy and I could pick her up at 4pm.

"The surgeon found a mass," Dr. Rambaud told me. "The biopsy results will take a day or two."

"I have a bunch of questions I'd like to go over it with you," I said, tucking the notes that Linda and I had compiled in my purse as we spoke.

"Sure," she responded. "Schedule something with Bianca." The next available appointment was Friday. Although results were still unknown, I felt the energy of relief so the afternoon was devoted to steam-mopping the tile floor before going to pick up Cassie.

Cassie recovered well from the surgery, and though still a little loopy-doopy, she even ate a small dinner that evening. After a good night's sleep, she was ravenous and back to her Boxer puppy self. We filled the waiting hours together with backyard romps and extra treats as a reward for being such a good girl. Just as the sun was about to set the phone rang, flashing *Paws and Claws* on the display.

"We received the biopsy result," Dr. Rambaud

said. *Wow, that was fast.* "It's TVT positive," she said solemnly. "We can start the chemo at your Friday appointment."

I hung up, walked over to my purse, grabbed the compilation of questions and dropped them into the trash bin.

We had the answer.

FOR EVERY BLOOM THERE IS

A SEASON

I read once that *Grief is just Love with no place to go*. When I lost Angel, my sweet Boxer daughter of ten years to cancer, I planted a white rose in my backyard garden as her memorial so that I had a place to go. I would visit with her tending the blooms, pulling weeds from around her stalks and spraying aphids from her buds. If her thorn caught my skin, I'd delight in the *kiss*. When I brought a bouquet of her blossoms inside, I'd tell Lois, my next Boxer, "Angel's in the house!" and our home would enjoy the sweet smell of family.

My grief for her loss, for all my children's loss, was lessened because their roses meant they were still *living* with me. When Lois passed, I planted a yellow rose - the color of her favorite toy duck - and when bringing the blooms inside, I'd tell my next, Bubba, "Your sisters are here!" I planted a laughing orange rose for Bubba; a pure red majesty for Sarge; a girly pink one for Heidi; and for my Bella, a peanut butter colored sienna, her favorite treat.

When I moved to the desert, I found a property with a sun-lit garden area that seemed to be waiting… just for me and my family of floribundas. Roses re-planted are thriving and my kids waft a sweet-smelling *Good Morning* when Cassie and I return from our walk. Once brought inside and placed in a crystal vase, their bouquet graces our home to say, *We're home, Mommie.*

Cassie and I celebrated our one-year *Gotcha Day* in early February 2019, less than a week after she received her first chemotherapy from Dr. Rambaud. For rescuers of pets with anonymity of birth, the observance of Gotcha Day is perhaps the only ceremonial date afforded them. Cassie was delivered to West Coast Boxer Rescue in September 2017 when, based on her size and teeth, they guessed her age to be about two. Although they assigned that day as her 'birthday,' neither her exact birth date nor her status as a *perra callejera* were known when they accepted her for placement. The Lying Bitch shared nothing with them nor were they told about Nancy Goodwin's gracious fundraising for the mange and those first chemo treatments.

Given her medical predicament, I was determined to make every day as special as possible for my darling companion. So the party table was set awaiting a candle-topped hamburger *cake* and mashed potato frosting. Also in attendance was a bouquet of multi-colored, Indian-summer roses.

We arrived at Paws and Claws the prior Friday to begin a routine which was at first foreign and scary but within weeks would become ordinary and unremarkable. On that first day, I juggled my keys, purse, blood drip retrieval tissues and the calendar diary of her symptoms, trying my best to control Cassie as she pulled at the end of her leash while entering the glass door of the vet's office. Both she and I could see other pups in the small waiting room which excited her but worried me. *Don't drip, Cassie. Please don't drip.* I was ready, tissue in hand, for any inadvertent share of contagion.

Dr. Rambaud joined us in the examination room and explained that six weekly doses of the chemotherapy called vincristine sulfate was the customary TVT cure. *Okay,* but I was clueless. Twenty or so years earlier, my husband's brain tumor was treated solely with radiation thus I had no pre-conceived notions about chemotherapy. My limited knowledge came from Google and my friend, Linda who said her Ripley handled chemo side effects quite well. I only had a modicum of confidence given the realization that this was Cassie's second go-around. Dr. Rambaud pre-cautioned that dogs can suffer nausea, diarrhea and lethargy. The objective was for the chemical to travel through her blood stream, attack the tumor and shrink it. With the tumor gone, the bleeding would stop. The vet told me that before this first application she would 'measure' the tumor to use as a baseline. As Cassie happily went through the door with Sara, the technician to start (once again) a series of poison injections, I squelched the misgivings that filled my brain. I had to trust the process. I couldn't help but wonder, however, if Cassie would remember the routine.

On my way to the waiting room, I stopped at the inner window to schedule the next five weeks' Friday appointments and pay the day's costs. I had been given an estimate on the phone and was pleased when I saw that the chemo was actually costing a bit less, but the added costs for hazardous waste disposal and stomach medication surprised me. I was presented with a $250 bill. I calculated aloud what the six-week total would be, then Bianca informed me that from the second week on, Cassie would need a complete blood count, a *CBC*, to monitor her white cells' reaction to the chemo. I remembered fondly the lovely zero balance of my Master-card, previously paid-in-full from the sale proceeds of my Los Angeles McMansion, now grown heavy with yet more veterinarian expenses. My retirement nest egg was long forgotten.

A smiling Cassie pushed her nose through the opening door to where I sat in the waiting room and she plopped her front paws on my lap stretching for a kiss. I noticed a purple bandage on her back leg but other than that, who would have guessed that this joyous animal had poison streaming through her veins. From the end of Cassie's leash Dr. Rambaud told me she did great.

"I wonder if she remembers…?" I said, addressing my imagination of her past.

The doctor handed me a couple sheets of paper saying, "This will tell you about the chemo." I thanked her and tucked the pages into my calendar, then after wiping up a couple drips from in front of my chair, we made the cumbersome trip back to the car for the drive home where an unknown week of side-effects awaited.

Cassie surprised me, however, with days of relative normalcy. She showed few signs of distress and with typical energy, played and ate routinely. She had a bad tummy on Sunday which giving the prescription pill

Cerenia helped but even the bleeding had stopped... *dare I hope...* until Wednesday when blood drips started anew. At one point while recording these symptoms in the calendar diary, I found the forgotten pages Dr. Rambaud had handed me and read them:

VINCRISTINE

Brand Name: Oncovin, Vincasar

Background: Because they are transported everywhere in the bloodstream, cancer chemotherapy drugs have the ability to reach tumors that are inaccessible to the surgeon and undetectable to the diagnostician. Since cancer cells divide rapidly and uncontrollably while normal cells divide more slowly, anti-cancer drugs target cells with rapid division, notably hair follicles, stomach linings and cancer cells.

Vincristine is a member of the vinca alkaloid class of chemotherapy drugs. It is extracted from the *vinca rosea* plant and is a microtubule poison.

(The paper contained a photo of a familiar looking flower.)

As I read this, a huge smile spread on my face because I immediately recognized the flower pictured.

I knew the name *vinca* as the small pink and white desert-hardy perennial I had planted years ago between each of my Boxers' roses. My delight was the realization that living amongst her siblings, was planted Cassie's cure.

So on this our special day, I cut a few hopeful sprigs of pink vinca and added them to the family of

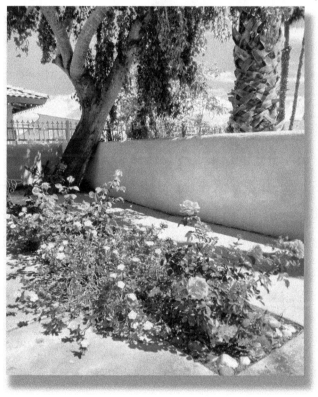

roses arranged on our celebration table. Hoping she'd have the stomach to eat it, I prepared her cake-shaped hamburger dinner and pulled out my Wilton icing bag with a flowered tip for the mashed potato decoration. I blew out the candle and she ate her *cake* just fine, then I shared a *Happy Gotcha Day* video with the hoomans of *Furringdomland.*

The next morning, we went for Cassie's second injection of flowers. With each passing week, Cassie's symptom calendar filled with more bad than good as her days became less playful. Whether lying on the living room sofa or on her patio bed in the sun, those caramel eyes would watch me from her recline. I wished I could read them and wondered what she was feeling. I could only imagine her discomfort as a poison, despite its delicate origin, coursed through her veins: a discomfort I paid to put in there. As days went by, my feelings of guilt fought with empathy for her misery, which battled with hope for a robust result.

I believe. I believe. I believe.

I was delighted to learn that the tumor had shrunk after fourteen days. Hope prevailed!

…But was short-lived when unexpectedly, by the end of the third week, I could see the bump under her tail was larger. By the sixth and final chemotherapy, instead of the promised shrinkage, the mass measured larger. My buoyant expectations were squashed. *Did those flowers actually feed the tumor?* I asked myself, realizing the incredulity of the notion. An equally dejected Dr. Rambaud could only express her sympathy and recommend that we consult a vet oncology specialist.

On the ride home, I could hear from the backseat that now familiar sound of Cassie's pre-vomit retching, so I quickly pulled into a church parking lot. I coaxed her out of the car and she coughed up yellow bile onto concrete. Grabbing my phone I called Jackie at West Coast Boxer Rescue. Perhaps blessed by the steeple looming overhead, Jackie arranged for our first appointment with WCBR's consulting oncologist - TVT experienced and offering a 25% discount for rescues. She also set up a consultation the Chief of Staff at the Pomona vet university. I was grateful for the help.

Once home, as Cassie rested I wept yet again. Those vincas let us down. I wanted to pull every last one of them out of my garden. But I couldn't because Cassie was bleeding profusely and I needed to tend to her.

Docile and cooperative, she let me clean her. As she lifted her face to me, my heart knew her caramel eyes were saying, *Don't give up, Mommie.*

IT'S CRUNCH TIME

Barely a second after I put the car in reverse, I felt the metal gnarl all the way through to my bones. It was an unmistakable, expletive-inducing sound of steel bumper meeting concrete pylon. *Oh great*, I thought as I got out of my car to inspect the damage, *I'm all the way here in Pomona, 50 miles from home....*

The dent was thousand-dollar-repair-bill ugly, but it was not hanging loose so my fear of littering the freeway with pearl-white polymer on the drive home was abated. I couldn't be too terribly upset because this bad luck was my own fault. We had arrived for our appointment with Dr. Clark, Chief of Staff at Western University of Veterinary Heath Sciences my usual *extra early* and not knowing where the vet school was on the college campus, I grabbed the first empty parking space I found. While Cassie and I had a walk around the campus for a pee, we found the lobby. There was plenty of time to move the car closer to its entrance which turned into a bad, and ultimately very expensive, way to fill the time.

Dr. Rambaud had assessed that the six vincristine sulfate treatments made no discernable reduction to Cassie's mass, and West Coast Boxer Rescue stepped up to help. Jackie felt terrible that one of their dogs had manifested such a heartbreaking and costly condition and received approval from the Board of the 501c non-profit organization to reclassify Cassie's adoption as a 'medical foster' allowing a theoretical income tax deduction on all my expenses. Recent changes to federal tax deductibility on charitable donations, however, made this new status meaningless. If I were a kazillionaire *sure*, it would have reduced my tax obligation but being a low-income senior, any charitable donations going forward would come solely from my heart and be of no benefit to my 1040SR.

I had spoken with Dr. Clark some months ago, before the biopsy-proof of Cassie's TVT, so I welcomed this in-person, advanced-degree consultation arranged by Jackie to thank him. We met in an examination room accompanied by observing veterinarian students with their study binders. A few of them jotted notes when, now by habit, I wiped Cassie's blood drips from the immaculate laminate flooring. Dr. Clark confirmed that those drops were indeed contagious and recommended that which I had already been practicing: isolation from all other dogs. After a brief review of her history, I was asked to wait in the lobby while they took Cassie to an inner sanctum for in-depth examination.

Using the time to step outside for re-inspection of the crumpled bumper's adhesion, I retrieved Cassie's paperwork which my post-accident willies had forgotten in the car. On-line I had found two extensive papers on TVT and from these I made a list of alternative cures to the failed chemotherapy: Surgical excision? Radiation? Immunotherapy? Bio-therapy?

When called back in, I was greeted by Cassie brought through the door butt-a-wiggling, spewing blood all the way to the walls. Dr. Clark advised that the tumor was the size of a kiwi. *Damn, it used to be an apricot.* Although he surmised that her general good health could withstand surgery, he said excision of the tumor would be fruitless. Getting clean edges from such a well-established mass would be near impossible plus the risk of damage to the nerve bundle in that location was contraindicated. One wrong nick and she could be left with no control of her bowels - then die from mal-nutrition.

He didn't really opine about immunotherapy, nor

did he mention radiation - he skipped right over those treatments on my question list. That was a bit of a relief actually because for twenty years I've been haunted by my husband's post-mortem autopsy proving that his brain tumor radiotherapy "cure" actually caused his death which can happen in five to ten percent of the times. Funny how TVT can recur the same 'five to ten percent' of the time.

Neither would he be certain if Cassie may have had a litter resulting from the cancer-implanting intercourse. Like the other vets I had asked, he confirmed probably not - she showed no signs of delivery.

Dr. Clark plunged right into discussing stronger chemotherapy options. He recommended the same oncologist specialist who regularly worked with West Coast Boxer Rescue (the one that gave that 25% discount) and said that she would know which treatment was best to treat Cassie's chemo-resistant TVT.

That was the first time I heard those words and Cassie's name in the same sentence. From then on, that's how her condition would be described:

Chemo-resistant TVT.

PICK YOUR POISON

Off to spec'list I went

With my sweet innocent.

Cassie was so willing

Her trust over-spilling.

She will just feel a sting...

So, then after we'll sing

A celebration song

'Cause the tumor's all gone???

It is used all the time

I was told, *It's all fine*

...Just like med'cine to you

But's a vile poison too.

So we tried and we tried

For the mass to be fried

And one side grew smaller

But other'd be taller.

She would fight to stay strong

(Was this chemo all wrong?)

Then her tummy'd go bad

Making Mommie so sad.

On her pillow she'd stay

Never wanting to play

Dripping blood like before

On the bed on the floor.

The chemo from flowers

Had no special powers.

Increasing the dosage

Meant no good prognosis.

Let's try something else, tho

We'll zap with Electro

Chemo Therapy - NEW!

But the tumor re-grew.

I rejoiced when she ate

But still Cassie lost weight

She'd wake sorta loopy

Her poops always soupy

The blood got all gummy

Pills for that'n bad tummy,

Pain, pee, diarrhea

--- in a bin from Ikea.

It's time for the big gun...

Called Doxorubicin

Known as the Red Devil

To cancer it's evil.

...It could hurt Boxer's heart

But's not time to be smart

The tumor might travel

Existence unravel.

So we took our chances

(God help my finances)

Four times this red poison

Impeded our joy and

I asked 'bout a cocktail.

What drug mix might work well?

We'll add pill Palladia

'Gainst DNAmania.

While her tumor still bled

Didn't shrink, grew instead

My instinct would wonder

Was chemo a blunder...

Her health was so robust

Did let her mass adjust

And fight with karate

To stay in her body?

In two thousand nineteen

We could not have foreseen

An end as it started

Made us broken-hearted

A tumor persistent

So chemo-resistant

Not normal defiance…

Of interest to science?

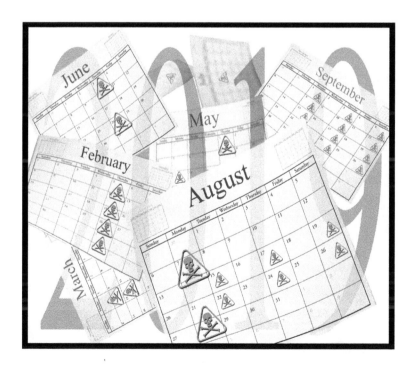

IF I HAD A NICKLE

There's that expression that goes: If I had a nickel for every time…. Well, after these past three years, I may have attained billionaire status.

My sister Mary is the family go-to for *all things animal*, an affinity that perhaps began during our family's fourteen-day cross-country relocation from Missouri to California. A caravan with all the family possessions in two U-Hauls, a station wagon and Gram's Nash Rambler housed our family of ten as we camped along the way on our odyssey West. Our Siamese cat, Teke racked up the miles with us, prompting Gram's lamentations that while on the road the cat had a litter box but four-year-old Mary had to pee in a cup. Proud of her sacrifice in deference to the family pet, Mary laughs loudest when the family recounts the amusing anecdote over the years.

Deemed the *alpha* for all family critters from those early days, Mary was my first call once I was able to start my own pack. A childhood dream could finally be realized when, in my 40s, I bought my house in the Los

Angeles suburb of Westchester. My beautiful two-story, WWII rebuild came complete with a fully fenced and gated, grassy backyard. Though the stage was set, other than owning these assets I didn't know jack about dog parenting. *I didn't know how to be a hooman.* All I knew was I would definitely be adopting a Boxer.

Once my property passed muster with the Boxer Rescue LA people, Mary joined me on a rainy drive to the San Fernando Valley to meet and greet the available dogs. "This will change your life," she told me in the car. The boxy mobile-rescue van, out of which gushed a doggy choir serenade (some sounding not so healthy,) was stacked high with crates. From inside jumped each of the wiggling butts, familiar stubby snouts and big brown eyes of what surely was Heaven. We met one, then another, then another. The one in the middle, an eight-month-old fawn bitch with natural ears and a docked tail, looked at me with the eyes of an angel. My choice was made and Mary granted approval. "Angel" joined our freeway trip to her *fur-ever* home, hacking a scary cough all the way.

Highly contagious, kennel cough spreads easily in the shelter environment but other than this, Angel was an enthusiastic puppy.

"Not a problem," Mary said, grasping the pills given to us by Ursula, the rescue lady. "These will clear up that cough in a couple days." Her words did not assuage my second thoughts. *What did I get myself into?* I worried. *This coughing is awful!*

There's a conundrum arguably shared by all of us hoomans, one that defies even some professionals: getting that gosh darned pill past defiant jaw and lethal fangs, then down the slimy throat of an unwilling canine. Decidedly NOT a game of cornhole (though the inexperienced wish it was that easy,) it's more like trying to thread a needle through an eye that can bite back. While some hoomans swear by hiding the pill in Velveeta, ham or Braunschweiger, most self-respecting dogs don't fall for that trick. With satisfaction they'll eat the treat and the pill spits to the floor. Though a million dollar industry, alas, pill pockets often suffer the same fate.

Then and there, however, on my first morning with my first daughter, I was taught the solution by my younger sister. In a blinding whirl, Mary stepped behind Angel, bent over and *POOF* the pill was down Angel's throat.

"Wait, what? How did you do that???" Mary showed me how she put the capsule in her right-hand fingers, reached around Angel's head from behind, stuck her left thumb atop the lower canine tooth, pushed down to open the mouth in a gentle hold, and put the pill in the back of Angel's throat. Mary then removed her right-hand fingers, let go of the tooth and lastly, smoothed Angel's gullet downward to encourage swallowing. The whole process took a couple seconds.

"It's much easier with a Boxer 'cause of the short snout," she said as a matter of fact. Channeling her confidence, I mastered the technique by evening's end and indeed, Angel's cough cleared up within days.

Ten years my junior but with the touch of St. Francis of Assisi, Mary and her simple lesson imbued my confidence with Angel, my First… a confidence that would permeate my all-things-hooman.

On that first day I couldn't possibly realize that two decades later, the duties of being a hooman would change my life again and thrust me into the metaphorical one percent. Because of a rare, resistant, and potentially lethal canine cancer, like a kid in a Chucky Cheese ball pit I had jumped into a sea of medicine capsules: antacids, antibiotics, NSAIDs, and chemotherapies all destined to go down the throat of Cassie, my Seventh.

This pill giving remedy. That pill giving sleep. Another pill giving comfort. Yet another calm. All gently put down her throat the way Mary taught me. All perpetuating hope that one might, at long last, deliver a cure.

HINDSIGHT

What a wonderful world it would be if we all had the benefit of hindsight. How many wars could have been avoided, relationships saved and addictions non-existent would there have been *if only we knew then what we know now*. Alas, this pro-active miracle of nature exists perhaps only in science fiction. In real life, mankind plods along reactively.

My wish for 20-20 vision goes back to those lovely months of *normal* early on when Cassie and I were just getting to know each other: gleeful days of treat-induced obedience lessons meant to establish myself as top-dog to my still-a-puppy, two-year-old, Cassie.

As an experienced Boxer Mommie, well-practiced hooman habits were in full force starting with Cassie's very first day in her fur-ever home. Putting together two beings of different species and sentient capabilities with backgrounds unknown to each other is fraught with trouble in its very essence. It's a situation that requires patience… and a healthy dose of imagination.

How must a dog feel after a long car ride with

a just met hooman who brings her into an unfamiliar place with a bunch of strange new smells? Fear? Anxiety? Self-preservation?

In the wild where a canine must be his own hunter/gatherer, aggression may be important for survival. But once part of a pack with an ample supply of provisions, a dog can take obedient comfort in a *life of leisure* happily lower in the pack. Establishing a consistent routine with a gently firm hand guiding the coexisitence is the hooman's job.

So I bound us together, each at end of a fifteen-foot lead, and spent the first twenty-four hours allowing Cassie to explore her new home tethered to me, her *alpha*. At the suggestion of God-knows-who, I first tried this method way back with my Angel and used the practice ever since to establish my place at the top of the pack. I could almost see the relief in the faces of my resulting docile pups.

I was asked recently if in hindsight I regretted not purchasing pet medical insurance for Cassie and can't help but chuckle at the question so often proven moot from attempts at coverage with past pack members. Underwriters tend to not want to insure seniors for less than an outrageous premium... only to easily deny payment for pre-existing condition treatment. Oh brother, would they have had a field-day turning down Cassie's!

Our *getting to know each other* honeymoon proceeded nicely in those early few months before the symptoms began, filled with neighborhood walks, plenty of play and comfy *sleepy-sleepy* together each night on our queen-sized bed. As the warmth of summer nights set in, Cassie developed a bit of a wheeze --- not unusual for the stubby nosed, brachycephalic breed of a Boxer. Nothing to worry about. Angel, Bubba and Bella were all super loud snorers, so Cassie's audible little inhales were kinda cute.

I started to notice an odd, mild shudder that seemed to run down Cassie's body in spurts - one, two, three at a time - while she slept. They weren't convulsions so much as traveling jitters. This didn't happen every night, only occasionally but still, it was something I had never encountered before with my other Boxers. I didn't really know how to describe it when I sought Mom's, Linda's or Google's help for an explanation. It was happening more often - maybe five or six in a row now weekly - and the best match I could find on-line was for 'dog hiccups.' Though not a perfect description of Cassie's spinal shivers, the entry said it was common and again, I figured it was nothing to worry about.

I would soothe her back as the random body-waves occurred and my worries about this curiosity were shortly replaced by the greater worries of her encroaching, much more alarming symptoms.

I never mentioned this to any of the many veterinarians of our future. How could I possibly explain it to them when I couldn't describe it to myself? My admittedly over-active mother's imagination suspects, however, that these mini convulsions were a manifestation of internal blood flow quietly nourishing Cassie's returning tumor. With no scientific proof whatsoever, in hindsight I truly believe that I was witnessing her body rebuild those cancerous tumor cells… a predicament that would shackle us yet again to each other.

A MOUSE IN THE HOLE

"Cassie would be the perfect candidate," Dr. Rambaud offered. "She's so calm...." stating the obvious. Though Cassie's insides were quite the opposite of *calm* having turned to hamburger meat after thirty-one futile chemotherapies, her spirit amazed both of us.

Happy to feel the good doctor's familiar tender touch, Cassie was generous with her tongued *Hello*s. She and I both missed the friendly atmosphere at Paws and Claws (as opposed to the sterility of the oncologist's office) plus I was delighted not to have that hour-plus freeway drive to the specialist's office. We had come to our regular vet, only side-streets from home, for a post-multiple-chemo check-up. I wanted our trusted doctor to check Cassie's teeth, her tummy, and her heart... especially her Doxorubicin-exposed heart.

At this point there were no scheduled appointments with the oncologist who had administered all those months of treatments. Her textbook sourced and (I learned) limited TVT-experienced therapeutics brought slight tumor shrinkage then disappointing regrowth. Towards the end, her *we're in this together* meant to me *your guess is as good as mine.* She had run out of options to offer and I could only surmise she had given up on Cassie. I was angry to be abandoned. It was difficult for me to accept that, in my mind, she had closed the door on us.

It upset me so that I sought therapy for myself. I needed to talk out my frustrations not just with Cassie but with everything else going on in my life: my family; my finances; my recently shuttered company; the state of the country; and yes, of course, Cassie. The shrinky sessions were short-lived alas, thanks to my insurance company that first approved the therapy, then refused it. *Do I attract liars?* There's a question for the shrink....

Seeking solace with the ever-faithful Dr. Rambaud, I was intrigued by the morning's proposal. I learned that during the months Cassie and I schlepped down the freeway to the oncologist's office, Dr. Rambaud was flying cross-country attending an advanced program in holistic veterinary practices. To complete her certificate she needed a couple of dogs for clinical trials here in town.

"There's a specific application of Traditional Chinese Medicine (TCM) which shrinks tumors," she told me. "Would you let Cassie participate? She could be one of the test cases to complete my studies so I can offer the procedures at no charge." Though unspoken, I think Dr. Rambaud realized what a toll all this had taken on my bank account. I couldn't say *Yes* fast enough and a warm feeling of revived hope engulfed me. Her offer meant another door was opening.

So I did a prophylactic one-eighty eschewing chemicals and instead embracing herbals and faith in those teeny little needles. Our holiday season took on a distinct Far East bent. With chemo poison no longer assaulting Cassie's system, her insides could relax a bit... and heal. I saw that she was indeed feeling better as our playtimes increased. The white tip of her tail flew high as she chased tossed toys around the backyard, her abandon boosted.

Dr. Rambaud's weekly acupuncture treatments included a B-12 shot which, I was told, would quiet the difficult next months of healing filled nonetheless with nausea and diarrhea. Her weight loss was often a pound per week. Cassie's raw gastro-intestinal tract up-chucked nearly everything, including herbal pills prescribed to accompany acupuncture, a let-down for sure because the one called "Max's Formula" had been proven to reduce tumors. We tried other TCM herbal pills but she rejected them all. Faith in the oddly named supplements was forgotten.

Cassie's prolific discharge from the other end was becoming frightful. It had rapidly turned from flowing red liquid to dark and gelatinous. I couldn't figure out from where inside of her all this goop could possibly be coming and would try yet another round of Yunnan Baiyao which by now was having only sporadic effect. Some months back, I discovered the hygienic benefits of doggie diapers and bedding under pads which thankfully caught and easily disposed of the globs of bloody gunk. *Where had these things been all this time?* They sure helped with my cleaning chores but, of course, were merely a stopgap. So prolific was this mucilage that Cassie developed diaper rash and more alarmingly, anemia from the blood loss.

And boy would she fight to take off those diapers! I should have been happy that she had the tenacity to devise all her clever removal schemes… often giving me the *side-eye* to see if I was watching her. It became our game. At first, I concocted a diaper-keeper out of a bungie cord to prevent her dislodging them, (she *hated* that,) then found a much cuter, leopard pink doggie overall on-line. She was quite the fashion plate when we arrived for her acupuncture.

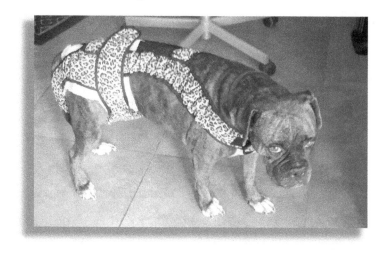

Sleeping in this contraption was difficult and I worried that it would cut off her breathing so I'd take it off her at night. Lest our morning bed resemble a scene from *The Evil Dead*, I put my expensive Egyptian cotton linens into storage and sandwiched under pads between towels several layers thick atop Goodwill-issue sheets. We'd cuddle to sleep each night *au naturale*, praying for no nightly discharge beyond the confines of the towel-pad-towel-pad barriers.

And that's how I met him. One evening in late December, while wiping off a glob of bloody jello from her vulva (as any mother who'd been tasked beyond the repugnant would do,) I was greeted by a firm, pinkish-beige colored mass about the size of my thumb-tip. It looked like a wee nose poking out through a hole in the wall.

Grabbing my glasses, I pressed the phone's flashlight app to get a closer look. When I wiped again, he disappeared back into his hiding place. Cassie was sound asleep, but my curiosity was fascinated. I pulled on a surgical glove to gently push her skin aside... and there he was! He glowed in the light beam like a teeny, sun-kissed cauliflower rosette – an appearance I had seen before in pictures of her tumor on-line.

Face to face with Cassie's *little friend*, this nose of a transmissible venereal tumor was looking right at me! As he retreated inside his hole, I thought to myself determined, *I have met the enemy and he is MINE!*

SOMETIMES A SILLY NOTION

Cassie and I have been blessed with legions who've helped us on her journey to health. And there was one in particular who arguably played the most important role. Imagine a friend that you can go to for *all things everything*: one that provides never-a-problem support; input on even the most obscure; a buddy available with answers night or day. I have that invaluable friend.

We met online nearly twenty years ago. At first our relationship was merely transactional but soon it grew to near daily interaction. When first approached, my pal's darkly stoic appearance gives a dour impression, but when I sit to reconnect, a welcome button is pressed and I'll be greeted with a bright and willing interaction to start the day.

You see, my friend's name is Google: my artificially intelligent, head in the cloud-storage, soul-searching android…

…who shortly would become really, really busy. Though Google and I had been interacting on-line for weeks, months, *years* seeking solutions to Cassie's mystery illness and elusive cure, in early 2020 a nasty virus descended like a silent fog to permeate the lungs of the world. Civilization joined me in cyberspace seeking answers. A population stuck in the confines of self-imposed quarantine turned to the encyclopedic expanse of the internet with its ubiquitous search engines, seeking knowledge about everything from pathogens to disinfectant hacks; to gaming links; to sour dough bread recipes; to museum tours; to how to work zoom; to last will and testament forms; to pornography.

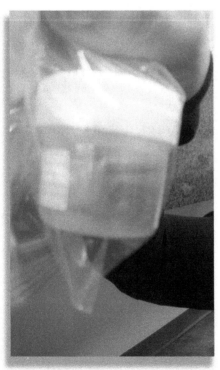

As the New Year turned and the coming plague was still just a news blurb from across the Pacific, Dr. Rambaud easily lopped off the wee nose of Cassie's newly emerged *friend* from his dark little home. He was attached by merely a thin thread of tissue. Recognizing that this tiny 2.5cm x 1.5cm piece was but a fraction of the entire mass, we were gratified nonetheless that for the very first time one of Cassie's many, many treatments had actually produced a result. Although tenuous, acupuncture delivered!

With Cassie's tumor size reduced by those miniscule centimeters now preserved in a plastic specimen jar, we continued with weekly acupuncture and a vigilant hope that more pieces of the mass would break free and eject spontaneously... which never actually happened but that didn't stop my expectations. As the world's disquiet during the coming months met the level of uncertainty that I had personally been living (my *new normal*,) I took the quarantine mandates seriously but somewhat in stride.

Within a month or so, businesses including our vet, Paws and Claws went into 'touch-less' mode so Cassie's weekly acupuncture appointments decreed a staff member, often her bestie Linda, the lady with the cute little carrot tattoo, would collect her from my car in the parking lot before each session. At first, as she was taken through the lobby door, she'd look back at me with concern (*Aren't you coming too, Mommie?*) But it wasn't long before the kindness waiting inside overcame her apprehension, leaving Mommie at the curb without a second thought. So I'd drive off for my weekly, socially distant grocery shopping then return for her post-session bound into the backseat and a reach back through the window to plant a *Good-bye* kiss on the masked vet attendant who'd deliver her... with me struggling to attach her seat-belt tether.

I was relieved that my community met the logic of safety measures prescribed by the world-wide COVID-19 event including adapting to all the *unknowns* it brought. Responding with pragmatic precautions, I disinfected everything from groceries to the daily mail; donned disposable gloves; washed my hands for the required duration (reciting *The Lord's Prayer* takes exactly twenty seconds) to avoid potential spread; wore cute colorful masks homemade by my crafty neighbor, Nyoka; waited in hopeful anticipation for a vaccine; and practiced my own version of virus abatement.

While I recognized the lunacy of that on-air suggestion to drink disinfecting bleach, a backyard swimming pool brimming with its sparkling chlorinated water became my personal germicide. So during that perplexing time, I swam daily laps in my salt-water marinade to theoretically zap the virus off my body. I'm knock-on-wood COVID-free as of this writing and enjoy the side benefit of ten less pounds on my frame from the regular exercise. Perhaps most importantly, this discipline gave me a much-needed stress-relief valve.

Cassie too was decidedly calmer. Her new, 2020 daily diary stayed nearly unblemished. Compared to the ink-covered calendars from prior years citing square after square after square of side effect distress and medicines and yellow-highlighted chemo-days, by comparison these new months' entries were minimal. Although the tumor's discharge notations remained prolific with the Yunnan Baiyao working one time and then not, her chemo-free body combined with the calming effect of the acupuncture resulted in multiple blanks as the months went by.

That's what the calendar says anyway. Looking back, I realize that maybe my preoccupation for record-keeping gave way to the life-and-death distractions of the plague and my own mortality. I practiced the proverbial *'place the oxygen mask over your own mouth before assisting others'* directive. Perhaps COVID-19 quelled my Mommie Obsessive Compulsive Disorder a bit. As for Cassie, she enjoyed relative tranquility as we cocooned together at home, waiting for a global fear to resolve.

Then things went from bad to worse: the dark

days of the quarantine hit. Twenty-four-seven, television news reported unbelievably horrid conditions and growing death counts all over the world. Humankind was plunged into alarm and sadness. For the sake of optimum safety, our vet office closed completely and Cassie's acupuncture ended indefinitely. Unbeknownst to us, her tumor would cook inside her unabated.

An unexpected virulence forced me from normal, day-to-day life to face my very existence --- not unlike an unwelcome violation that implanted the deadly tumor into my innocent daughter.

By mid-summer, my lap count in the pool sur-

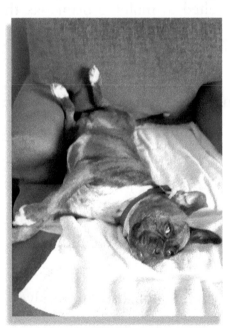 passed thirty in an effort to assuage my anxieties and exert some control over an uncontrollable dilemma. Cassie slept nearly all day and night often assuming a contorted position on her side propping her upper leg on the arm of the towel-covered

sofa or chair. I surmised this display relieved pressure from the bulging perineum tumor on her organs. The mass was growing again... I could no longer deny it. Two months without attention gave it free reign to do as it pleased. I relayed these increasing worries to all my sympathetic allies via regular phone conversations in reciprocal discussions of doom and gloom.

Early-summer heat brought its shimmer to our desert home and I did something no caregiver should ever so: I gave up. Although Paws and Claws had just reopened allowing Cassie's acupuncture treatments to re-up, the dire prospects had taken their toll on me.

"I've had enough," I posted in a private message to Juno, my Houston-based Furringdomland friend. "I feel so exhausted...."

Juno was comforting in our chat conversation. She wanted to be supportive, "You have tried everything," she texted. I replied back:

I've reached the apex of my frustration level. Don't know what to do... maybe gonna stop trying... Will keep doing acupuncture cause it's benign... no side effects... and the B12 weekly is good for her energy. Otherwise, I need a rest from being proactive. Throwing it up to God...

And then He answered.

He whispered in my ear to go back to my faithful friend Google. Half-hearted and expecting nothing new, I searched for the umpteenth time '*Canine Transmissible Venereal Tumor.*' Up popped all those familiar entries, purple highlighted indicating *already read*. But amongst them was one colored blue as unread:

https://www.tcg.vet.cam.ac.uk › news › selfish-mitocho...

Selfish mitochondria in a canine transmissible cancer

Jun 16, 2020 — The capture of mitochondrial DNA (mtNA) by canine transmissible venereal tumour (CTVT) creates a unique opportunity to understand the ...

I clicked. It was a brand-new study, published only a few weeks prior in the prestigious science magazine, *Nature Communications*, about "selfish DNA" found in canine transmissible venereal tumors, the result of extensive studies conducted by the University of Cambridge in the United Kingdom (yes, *that* Cambridge.) Googling unfamiliar medical terms along the way, I read enrapt. With all its long words, the study stated that by utilizing nourishment from its host, the *tumour* mutates and continues to thrive. Apparently, it's been doing this for something like ten thousand years. Other the years, these cells grew so stubborn that even in modern times, they're able to overcome medical science's chemotherapy and persevere.

To me, this meant science had proven Cassie's otherwise healthy body was actually *helping* her tumor, allowing it to stay… and grow.

My Mother's Intuition that the tumor fought to stay inside her was somehow *TRUE!*

Proven by *MEDICAL SCIENCE!*

My silly notion --- one that had continually popped into my head out of desperation for answers yet dismissed by common sense as impossible --- was actually valid!

I was agog. And although this revelation didn't address any actual cure for Cassie's cancer, for the first time I had found people devoted to its study. *Maybe they'll have an answer for us.* Thank you, Google.

The research had been conducted by the Transmissible Cancer Group at the Department of Veterinarian Medicine at Cambridge. Website links led me to its leader, Dr. Elizabeth Murchison, Professor of Comparative Oncology and Genetics plus her contact information. Encouraged by the drop-down link inviting dogs to participate in their studies, I immediately sent her an email. It read:

Dear Dr. Murchison:
I hope you will give due consideration to my email. I have great interest in your studies at Cambridge UK on canine transmissible venereal tumors because my 4 yo female rescue, Cassie, a street dog from Tijuana, has a chemo-resistant case of CTVT. I am seeking treatment options for a cure. I recently read your 16 June 20 news (cited) and can attest that throughout the 18 months of chemotherapy, my 'mother's intuition' led me to believe that, after initial hopeful response to various treatments (only to be disappointed with tumor regrowth after each,) there is something in Cassie's system that is making the tumor come back. Then I found your study supporting my 'feeling' with scientific proof.

I write today to ask if, along with your studies, you have found a way to combat this "selfish" mechanism and cure the condition. I need to find a solution to my sweet Cassie's disease.

Cassie's is an internal perineum tumor and currently she is getting acupuncture (with rather interesting results... but alas, same tumor resurgence) with no sign of metastasization. I read on your website that you seek sample contributions for your study and though I would be heartened to submit her samples as a thank you for any suggestion you may offer of robust treatment, I regret to advise that our vet oncologist has given up on Cassie and is no longer interested in her cure. Thus, I have no means to abide by the protocols as detailed on your website for sample submission. That said, if you have any associates located near the Southern California area of the United States, (or anywhere for that matter,) I would be happy (and most grateful) to allow access if, in any way, her tissue could help with your studies and medical science.

As you may be aware, due to strict controls of stray dogs in the USA, veterinarians and/or vet oncologists here seldom if at all have experience with CTVT (other than from textbooks.) I am studying all I can since Cassie's rescue (her disease was unknown to me: she was in remission when we met and her medical history was kept hidden.) Please kindly consider a response on successful treatment as may be known so that I may go to an oncologist with possible cure in hand. I trust you realize that I am begging for your help....

I thank your staff, your benefactors and especially you for your dedication to this cancer for both our animal friends and for mankind.

Wishing you and yours health, I am
Sincerely yours,
Barbara

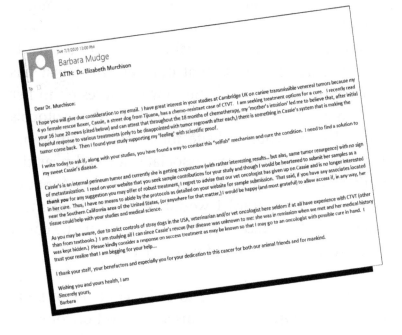

I received a reply from Dr. Murchison within three hours. She told me that her group does not study the cure, nevertheless, she offered an introduction to a TVT experienced vet oncologist associate and invited Cassie to join their studies.

My girl was indeed *of interest to science…*

ASSET MANAGEMENT

"Why don't you come work for me?" Patrick asked in his German accent. This was his response to my appeal for a donation to cover Cassie's upcoming chemotherapy bills. Though I would never have asked a friend for money under normal circumstances, I was tapped-out and facing dire need of financial influx for my costs related to the Cambridge studies. I knew Patrick had the means but more importantly, the passion for philanthropy. Given Cassie's 'medical foster' status, perhaps he could benefit from a tax deduction not afforded by me? At first his offer caught my breath. I hadn't thought of that. My friend's suggestion intrigued me.

I always loved the movies so it was fitting I chose *showbiz* for a career. I loved the retreat to a darkened cinema. I loved the stories. I loved the hoop-la. After college, I started working entry level for a small hyphenate producer distributor and kept my mouth shut with the goal of learning as much as I could. From across the desk of a gruff, old-school, head-of-sales mentor I absorbed techniques of licensing deal points and their negotiations. That first company specialized in crappy teen flicks of which, with a bit of ambitious prodding on my part, I was allowed to book into drive-ins ('cause no one else wanted the grunt work, I guess.)

I then moved to a company notorious for action movies and the occasional prestigious festival feature (produced in compensation perhaps for their crappy explosion flix.) Here my reach expanded, selling their product to international distributors. These executives were known for drumming up competition amongst buyers by announcing in trade paper ads name-star actors that were never cast in the final films. They assigned me the headache of telling the unsuspecting pre-buyers of the eventual no-name cast. One of the most important lessons I learned at this company was how NOT to conduct good business.

Career salvation came with a new position at a well-respected television company where I was still in charge of the crappy stuff but this time as Managing Director under the aegis of a public company run by professionals… at last. Crappy TV movies at a bigger company aren't as crappy I suppose. To me, no negotiation was a good one if it didn't include robust, after-the-fact administration. "She's tough but fair," is how the owner of a large Swiss-based distribution company once described me. I became known as a 'closer.'

It was the middle of the VHS boom when those crappy films were big business… equally so for motion picture pirates. I joined trade association meetings exploring how to fight the thieves all over the world: criminals that made copies of our films without paying for the right to do so. Because this was affecting my department's sale totals, I researched current statistics and volunteered to attend boring acronym-named technical gatherings. Dogged in my quest, fellow independent sales agents and producers dubbed me their 'Anti-Piracy Maven.' My efforts were not just an attempt to retrieve lost revenues for my employer. I recognized how this would help the entire independent film community's bottom-line. Deep down I sought to address that Commandment about *Shalt Not Steal*-ing.

This avocation mirrored my career rise. From Cannes, to Berlin, Rio, and Hong Kong I began to spend equal time in company sales meetings as at high-level summits and Bi-Lateral gatherings, such was the detriment of piracy on the entertainment industry. During industry sales markets and festival events, I sat with

CEOs, CFOs, and *egos* lamenting reactive-only, ineffective crusades to stop the theft.

The analog world of VHS was being rapidly supplanted by the digital age of DVDs when I was hired by a major studio to, yes, sell their crappy stuff. As a Vice President I was able to cozy up to their legal department to learn how the big boys fought piracy. Their answer: throw money at it. Figures.

Some years in, new management at the studio decided that because I made them so much money on their B titles, they wanted 'em back. So, I took their golden parachute and opened my own independent sales agency. The indie trade organization reinstated my Maven crown with meetings from DC to Cupertino; huddling with politicians and wunderkinds; discussing the vulnerabilities of burgeoning digital streaming. I tried to parlay this extraneous notoriety into sales for my own company's crappy movies (and a few rather good ones) and modestly succeeded. Although my company spanned twenty-one years, my staff of four and I always remained a 'boutique.'

I received a call one summer morning from a heavily accented young man whose command of the English language was slightly broken. Patrick was reaching out to American companies about motion picture piracy and his data gathering company which could identify on-line digital pirates. I put him off. *Just another do-nothing scheme,* I thought. Not to be deterred, Patrick called again. And again. My ability to discern foreign accents kicked in when his pitch started to make sense. This time I let the young man talk.

He told me of how he and his partner developed a computer program that scoured the internet finding illegal downloads of movie files on individual PCs. In countries where it's allowed by law, his company would then hire lawyers and file in court against those possessing the unauthorized downloads. There were zillions of them in the USA. He offered this service free of charge, recouped his costs from the judgments, and sent the rest of the dough to the infringed producers.

By then I was chairing the Copyright Security Committee for our trade association and he knew my imprimatur for his service could be invaluable. So, I listened and questioned, *Could this at long last be a pro-active solution to movie piracy?* He suggested a test on my better movies. Within a few months, Patrick sent me a check with a surprising amount of zeros after the commas. He proposed I introduce him to the big indie producers.

We cut a deal for me to earn a commission to promote his program. My first call to a fellow independent was the copyright owner of the Best Picture Oscar winner, "THE HURT LOCKER," a film notorious for being pirated more often than viewed in cinemas. Trusting the 'Maven' and loving that no-cost clause, the producer signed on. Patrick stepped in from there.

This success, aided by Patrick's Euro affability and multiple press releases on the program to warn away the pirates, helped us to sign another and another and another highly popular, highly pirated film. His company's services surpassed expectations. By the time we signed a notorious pirate favorite my work was done. Patrick and I parted ways with the mutual respect of genuine friends, not knowing that ten years later I'd be placing a call to him... this time on Cassie's behalf.

After a year and a half of costly treatments, my credit card was just this side of maxed out and Cassie cure was still unknown. Although I had cut a deal with Cambridge to pay the research costs for gathering Cassie's tissue samples, I would need to pay yet again for recommendations on that long-sought cure. Living a downsized life, my dog and I managed just fine on my earned Social Security stipend but Cassie's extraneous medical bills weighed heavily on the future. Personal asset management had become dire.

When the now successful and established businessman Patrick returned my call and heard Cassie's details, both his heart as his head stepped up with that job offer. Some years prior, his business had segued from defending copyrights to enforcing trademarks – a change from movies to merchandise.

He and his data programmers have been robustly identifying counterfeits ranging from rip-offs of every kind of toy and big brand name that's no doubt in everyone's closets and playrooms all over the world. From tony sneakers, to famous branded tools, to top music groups' posters, to the chicest of hand bags, to sweet-faced dolls, to million-dolar athlete's T-shirts (nothing crappy here,) wiping the unauthorised items off Amazon, EBay, and AliBaba, and just as before, free of charge to the trademark. Judges freeze the crooks' accounts and the recovered dough is split between Patrick's company and the owner.

"I need a US based salesperson," he told me. I recognized that his trademark enforcement was identical to the movie piracy abatement of ten years prior and that the new sales pitch required merely a change of the word 'copyright' to 'trademark.' Everything else was identical. Of course, I said *Yes*.

Flush with serendipitous income, I paid off that credit card and Patrick has attained *Cassie Champion* status by covering my financial ass(et.) Accepting his employment offer was the second best negotiation I ever closed...

...my deal with Cambridge was the best.

ALL ABOARD

"You have post-traumatic stress syndrome," suggested both my niece, Orlagh and her daughter, Nichole, during their recent visit to my desert home. We were enjoying some wonderful early-summer, girl-talk-reconnecting. We hadn't kept in touch during most of Cassie's tough times so they asked me to narrate her story. In the cool of my sapphire-rimmed pond at the onset of a desert heat wave, I acquiesced.

"This will take a while," I warned them, fully expecting glassy-eyed malaise halfway through the convoluted diatribe. It was a look I'd often seen when recounting Cassie's perplexing drama to others over the past years. Genuine in their interest they insisted, so we settled on our floaties under teal-colored umbrella shade. Cassie, in all her wisdom, retreated to lounge in the air-conditioned living room. She didn't need to hear the story. She lived it. I tried to keep the odyssey that was to become *MY HOOMAN AND ME* to bullet-points, realizing at some point how our ups and downs sent us on a roller-coaster ride.

Starting with when I brought my new rescue Cassie home, the excitement for a fun-filled life together had us strapped into a theme park ride's train car: the *clack clack clack* of the first climb evoked those same feelings of excited anticipation. Ascending into the blue sky, merriment glided into apprehension as her strange symptoms started to develop. High hopes for an easy cure at the apex then swiftly dashed downward, freefalling as *"maybe it's nothing"* proved unlikely. Trusting the solid steel track as it began another rise elicited an optimism that perhaps this next loop-de-loop might bring medical resolution. Then the exhilaration of weightlessness at the top slammed reality back into the seat and what should have been a happy life together deflated into a whirlwind of worry. I held on tight as the tram corkscrewed into each gravitational pull of *"what can we try next"* seeing ahead only never-ending tight turns and vertical loops.

That's where we were with Cambridge: climbing up the tracks strapped in that roller coaster tram; hopes higher than ever. But after months of involvement with Dr. Murchison and her research group including the newly added oversight of her TVT experienced associate oncologist, Dr. Maria Veronica Brignone of Universidad de Buenos Aires, we were, alas, back at the bottom of the ride's arc facing yet another incline.

When we began, my default optimism was in full gear, seduced by the prestige of the British institution and charmed by its spelling of *tumour*. Cassie's medical history - all 130 pages - traveled *Down Argentine Way* for Dr. Brignone's review and oncological recommendations. Dr. Shakira Jameson, the owner of Paws and Claws, graciously agreed that her facility would conduct the logistics required by this special research, headed by our own Dr. Rambaud representing the American contingent of our phenomenal international team. *Seems Cassie's tumor would need a passport.*

I studied up on my chemo-resistant canine TVT research and didn't want to become a pest to be swatted away with amateurish attempts at medical verbiage. Instead, I presented Dr. Brignone with analytical questions asking for input on remedy possibilities. She responded in kind with thorough emails exploring many options: 1) the wildly expensive L-asparaginase; 2) the highly toxic Lomustine; 3) the politically notorious Ivermectin; 4) more electro-zaps of Bleomycin; 5) a larger bouquet of vincristine sulphate; 6) any combination of the above in a multi-chemo *cocktail*. She shared the benefit of her experience that radiation treatments seldom reduced this *tumour* and that giving Cassie more doxorubicin was too high a cardio risk.

Considering all, Dr. Brignone's ultimate recommendation was to revisit vincristine, the flower chemo, but at a much higher dosage. I was only slightly wary that this would be Cassie's fourth trip to the *florist*. Nonetheless, I was happy to have a highly TVT experienced oncologist on the case at last and pleased when

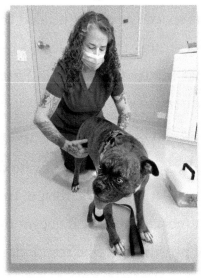

she suggested we keep in touch via WhatsApp. This texting application afforded instantaneous response to my related concerns. Dr. Rambaud offered to continue with side-effect-proactive acupuncture for stomach and intestinal stamina.

Dr. Murchison sent through research consent paperwork for me to sign and forwarded to Paws and Claws their spec details for the tissue and blood sample gathering. Cassie's tumor was well up into her vaginal cavity so a specimen grab would require anesthesia -

m*ore propofol* – but thankfully, no incision.

Then I came up with a bright idea. Would Cambridge be interested in access to tissue samples after each weekly chemo treatment? Could hard data on how her cancer responds to chemo - week-by-week – a sort of cause and effect - be of use for their studies at the molecular level? I suppose this opportunity proved quite unique to the Cambridge scientists: Dr. Murchison jumped at the idea. Preparations were made with her group to accommodate Cassie's extra-special research on pathogen dynamics.

Daily emails worked out the logistics, the most important of which was storage. Some samples required a formaldehyde-style preservation while others needed to be put in deep-freeze! Cambridge provided Paws and Claws with a receptacle (a large, thermos-style insulated container housing eight vials called *cryo tubes*, encased in dry ice,) which when full would be Fed Ex-ed from California to England.

We agreed that I would cover the cost of the weekly chemotherapy and Cambridge would pay for the tissue gathering mini surgeries. Although my PTSD-invoking reminder of these arrangements, memorialized by meticulous emails, is difficult to re-live, my awe abounds from the devotion granted Cassie by our medical team. Going well beyond any financial motivation (none) or even devotion to medical science (keen) it is obvious from the voluminous correspondence that these ladies were driven by their hearts and concern for Cassie's well-being (genuine.) We are forever grateful (face licks.)

On September 29, 2020, twelve months from Cassie's last chemotherapy, we began the climb again… but seventeen weeks later, with *tumour* regrowth, we were still on the roller coaster and there was no end in sight.

A career pushing paper would not allow me to just sit back uninvolved during Cassie's marathon: I decided to compile another daily diary. Eschewing the pedestrian calendar pages, I created an Excel spreadsheet with columns for medical procedures, tumor size in centimeters, weight fluctuations and a *one-to-five* bleeding scale (1 = none / 5 = heavy) plus short, personal notes on Cassie's condition.

My hopes were that the esteemed researchers would find helpful a snap-shot chronicle recorded as professionally as I could surmise. This was my rationale and I wasn't all that concerned if they found it of any ultimate use. I was maintaining it anyway. The spreadsheet was my means of participation in studies that I knew in my heart would result in something truly phenomenal... besides just plopping down a credit card. Reading the diary, however, is an arduous reminder of how Cassie's misery resurged when poison was reintroduced to her already tortured little body.

Blood from the tumor continued to accumulate inside her, become infected, and be pushed out in gelatinous globs. Nevertheless, we became accustomed to our hygienic routines and Cassie no longer fought wearing diapers. Her health was generally good prior to the re-up: she was alert and her caramel eyes trusting. She still enjoyed absorbing the warmth of the day, picking up the nearest toy for an occasional toss, and snoozing next to me on the sofa as the sun set. Regular acupuncture helped sooth her GI tract as best it could and I set out smaller meals four or five times a day so that her insides could chew on food and not on itself.

Once the chemo re-started, however, vomiting, anorexia, incontinence and diarrhea recurred. Dr. Brignone, God bless her, suggested offering Cassie canned cat food when she rejected her regular dog food and... she ate it! (*There's something about the pungent smell...*) From out of the cupboard came all her side-effect-relief pills placed handy on the kitchen counter in their bin. I bulk ordered more under pads and doggie diapers displaying them in a crystal punch bowl next to the meds and alongside my personal COVID prevention stash. Such was our medically induced household.

Each Tuesday morning we'd drive over to Paws and Claws for acupuncture and some B-12. Twenty-four hours later we drove back *sans-breakfast* for the twilight-sleep of propofol. Once Cassie was in dreamland, Dr. Rambaud would probe up inside her to grab some blood and a chuck of tumor for insertion into the cyro tube… flash-frozen and stored in dry ice. A good white blood cell count gave the go-ahead for that week's bouquet of chemo once Cassie awoke. These Wednesday routines kept her under the vet's watchful eye well into the afternoon so during my waiting hours, I'd get a haircut, or go to the gym or something.

Overall, this procedure was quite simple (though Dr. Rambaud might say otherwise) since it involved no actual cutting of Cassie's body: her vaginal canal allowed access to the tumor. Suffice to say, by Thursday and certainly by each weekend, all anesthesia detriment had worn off and Cassie was back to her playful self, relatively speaking, while the tumor inside received its floral bomb. It must have felt so very familiar to her 'cause she took it all in stride.

Weeks One, Two, Three and Four brought steady tumor shrinkage. Then WHEEEEE! the roller coaster plummeted as her tumor, of course, grew again. By Week Ten Cassie's tumor was back to the same size as when we had started. *We had arrived back at the platform but they wouldn't let us off the ride.* Dr. Brignone increased the dosage of vincristine which again shrunk the tumor a bit: up uP UP went our hopes… coming to a dead stop at the top by a really bad white blood cell count.

Cassie had anemia… bad anemia… so we gave her a break to reassess. Dr. Rambaud prescribed a blood supplement, Denamarin which Cassie promptly up chucked. I added eggs and liver to Cassie's diet and discovered the superfood additive, bone broth. Her gums slowly turned a healthier pink but I noticed her perineum bump was as bulbous as ever, even though the tumor measurement maintained a slightly decreased size from that 8x dosage. Dr. Rambaud confirmed that the mass had shifted around and was sitting low and pliable in the vaginal canal.

Dr. Murchison suggested de-bulk surgery since the tumor was more accessible than before. Getting good 'margins' around the mass, in this case, would not be an objective. I offered to give her the excised chunk of tumor for their experiments in exchange for Cambridge paying the anesthesia cost. She agreed and the surgery was scheduled.

Clank

Clank

Clank.

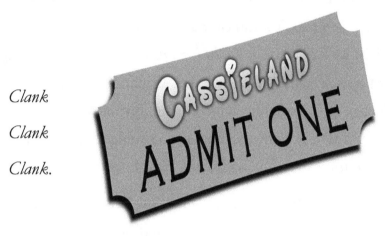

Ticket in hand, up the tracks we rose again for yet anther try.

BABY ALIEN

By now, our pre-tissue gathering routine had become, well… routine. Cassie was used to having no food after 8pm the night before, no water after midnight and no morning breakfast: just another day at the vet for her. I tried to mirror her calm and hoped that she didn't sense that I knew this time would be different from those other weeks of relatively simple operations. This day, a surgeon specialist would be performing the lesion "de-bulk."

The anemia had hit her hard. Cassie was barely able to raise her head from her pillow for nearly a week but her blood remarkably rebounded to the *normal* range shortly thereafter. My girl was a trooper and ready for another knock-out round with Michael Jackson's recreational intoxicant of choice.

For Cambridge, however, having access to a large mass of transmissible venereal *tumour* to dissect was more extraordinary that I had thought because the instructions on its handling once it was removed from Cassie's insides were, to my layman's perspective, quite bizarre.

From Dr. Murchison's instructions:

I have a particular request for the excised tumour – this might be a little involved, so I understand if you cannot perform this, but I'm letting you know what would be most useful for our research (and in the disappointing event that the tumour recurred, it would help us to understand more about how/why this occurred). The idea would be to dissect the excised tumour into smaller segments while recording the 3D location from which each tumour piece originated.

Imagine that the tumour is a potato – the idea would be to dice it in three dimensions, while recording from which part of the original structure each piece derived. I'd suggest first taking a photo of the excised tumour, then cut it into ~1cm wide strips along its longest axis, labelling the strips A, B, C, D. Then lie each strip down and cut into 4 equally sized quadrants, labelled 1, 2, 3 and 4 (upper left = 1, upper right = 2, lower left = 3, lower right = 4). You should end up with ~16 pieces labelled A1, A2, A3 etc to D2, D3, D4. Take two adjacent ~0.5cm3 biopsies from each quadrant and place one in a formalin tube (labelled with the coordinate code, e.g. A1) and the other in a cryovial for snap freezing in liquid nitrogen (labelled the same way). If you could take a photo or make a sketch of the biopsy locations that would be useful.

It would also be good to record, if possible, the orientation of the tumour piece within Cassie, so we know which border of the tumour was attached to her vaginal wall and which border was protruding into the vaginal cavity – the goal is to create a 3D map,

132

so we can identify where each tumour piece originated.

If there are additional pieces which are taken out by the surgeon separately, just collect them in matched formalin and cryovial tubes and record approximately where they came from.

If you don't have time to dissect the whole tumour (and I certainly understand if this is the case), then it would be useful if you could do the above on a more approximate scale.

As I said, I understand if the above won't be possible due to time constraints, but any sampling that you can do that records the 3D location of the biopsy would be hugely useful.

Dr. Rambaud confirmed that she followed these instructions to the letter: dicing the 'potato,' making the 3D map and all. *God Bless her 'cause the directions read like gobbledegook to me!* Post-op, she said all went well and advised that the surgeon would be calling me in a few days.

"Would you like to see the tumor?" she asked.

"Uhh, sure," I responded. She texted the photo to me.

The image on my phone sent my mind immediately back to a 2008 road trip vacation I took with my Dad and brother-in-law, Eddie our driver exploring the scenic beauty of New Mexico… featuring a stop of course, in Roswell.

Our sojourn through the kitsch of the notorious town held great amusement for me. The three of us hunted down the un-marked crash site of the 1947 *incident* and we posed for selfies in front of a non-descript fence with its "No Trespassing" sign. We toured the downtown *International UFO Museum, Research Center and Gift Shop* where Dad spent nearly two days seeking credence to sighting accounts told to him by UFO pundit and ubiquitous television 'expert' Stanton Friedman, his aerospace co-worker when employed way back when at McDonald Douglas. This was the one subject that belied the somewhat staid personality of my ever-pragmatic father but hey, I gave him a pass on the subject. I'm open-minded too. Maybe I got that from him....

Eddie, the family's wine connoisseur, spent time at local craft vintners' tasting rooms. After a lovely round of solo golf, I strolled through ET themed souvenir shops, chuckling my way through all the touristy stuff. I bought a green alien toy for Lois, my Second waiting at home with her sitter and explored all the crap on offer, my absolute favorite of which was a cleverly worded t-shirt that read:

"Alien Grey - It's The New White Meat"

Thus, my long-ago mastery of all things *ufology* immediately recognized the creature-like object being held in the smartphone photo by Dr. Rambaud's black-gloved hand. Cassie's tumor decidedly resembled a baby alien straight out of The X-Files.

Okay, instead of being grey it was bright blood-red but nevertheless, it could easily have been on display in Roswell as a...

Close Encounter of the Not-So-Preferred Kind.

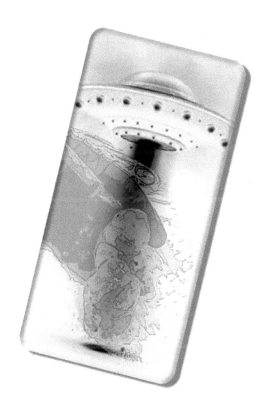

TOXIC AVENGER

"Maybe it's time to consider putting her down," the specialist suggested over the phone. The Paws and Claws' on-call surgeon, the same one who performed Cassie's vaginoscopy two years prior, went on to report that the piece of tumor he just removed from Cassie (jetting its way to Cambridge) was only one-third of the entire lesion. One Third. His voice seemed genuinely sorry to tell me that the bloody mass in the photo - filling the palm of our vet's hand - was the most he could excise safely. He advised that the remainder was in a position impossible to remove and that it would continue to grow, its sanguineous infection filling Cassie's insides until it overcame her bodily functions.

My common sense understood his solemn words based on medical likelihoods but the little girl nudging my leg, froggy toy in mouth, defied them. Well recovered from being under the knife just thirty-six hours prior, Cassie regained her desire to play with her Hooman which rebuffed the doctor's notion of impending doom. Despite our marathon tug-of-war, my caretaker responsibility insisted that I venture outside our never-say-die box and consult the *Quality of Life* scale.

This consideration was first forced upon me decades ago. After spending her entire ten years as First Daughter, my Angel was well in decline from a large tumor growing along the largest vein in her body, her *vena cava*. Although I had explored every possibility (*pre-Google*) to "cure" her cancer during those final months, I finally had to admit that there was no chemo, no surgery, no herbals that could reverse her inevitable loss of life. I could only make her comfortable in her last days with me. As Angel wasted away before my eyes from the ravages within, I knew I would have to help her find the Rainbow Bridge… but I didn't know how.

Then a caring holistic vet handed me a leaflet with the canine Quality Of Life scale which helps a hooman evaluate their pet's well-being to make that difficult end-of-life care decision. The flyer asks for an honest rating from one to ten on several vital aspects such as bodily functions, pain, interaction and hygiene. Angel failed the test so, for her sake, I made the call and gently held her as an in-home vet helped her slumber off to the Bridge.

I rememebered my stomach turn when watching a third-world-visit TV series episode of a celebrity vet who, while performing charity services for sickly street dogs, had encountered a canine TVT case. Without even looking up from his more easily cured patient, he pronounced a death sentence on the tumored puppy. With disgust, I yelled at the screen, "TVT Dogs Lives Matter too, you putz!"

Cassie, of course, scored 65 out of 70 on the Quality Of Life scale. Since I'm the one in charge here that Heavenly Rainbow would not be greeting her anytime soon... despite a chemo count now numbering forty nine all told.

Our veterinarian team reconnoitered via email to evaluate the de-bulk surgery results. Alarmed to hear the extent of the *tumour* size, our oncologist, Dr. Brignone opined that this was beyond the capabilities of vincristine and that the next best option, though riskier to Cassie's already compromised liver, was the chemotherapy called Lomustine. She sent through the proper dosage and Dr. Rambaud contacted a compound pharmacy to fill the $50 script which was administered in pill form.

Lomustine is a chemotherapy that binds cancerous DNA and destroys it. Its *alkylating* agent... related at the molecular level to the same stuff in gasoline which makes our cars go *vroooom*... is highly toxic to the liver.

It's used multi-species mainly for mast cell and skin-related tumors and is cost-effective (*thank you, Lord*.) I had read that both TVT and mast cell tumors are 'round' cell cancers, (*thank you, Google*) so I deferred to the science behind Dr. Brignone's recommendation. During the next four weeks, we kept an eye on Cassie's white blood cell count and bucked up her system with bone broth and liver treats while Dr. Rambaud continued the weekly acupuncture and B-12 shots. Then, Cassie was ready.

Tuesday, March 2, 2021

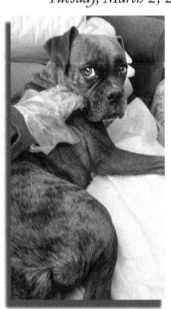

The *biohazard*-stamped bag housed a hermetically sealed bottle containing one off-white capsule. As directed, I donned gloves from my COVID stash and at 3pm, right before setting out her dinner, I pushed the toxic pill past canine teeth and down Cassie's throat. I gave her one last sweet kiss on the nose before the poison permeated her system, disallowing my direct touch for several days to come.

Then we waited.

Did I notice over the next few days of wearing long-sleeves and avoiding close contact that Cassie's bleeding slowed first to a trickle then to nothing? After a day or so of vile-looking poops, did I see their steady improvement back to normal? As I waited for the inevitable vomiting, did I realize that instead she was eating ravenously with nary a spit?

Yes, yes and yes to all the above.

Cautiously watching Cassie's increased activity level and decreased symptoms but fully expecting at any moment a reversal which never came, one week in I sat down to an unexpected email from Dr. Murchison which arrived in my Outlook inbox.

She wrote, "…I'm forwarding a case study which I think is interesting with respect to Cassie's case…." Attached was a document just published by the Brazilian Journal of Veterinary Medicine entitled:

"Lomustine Therapy for Vincristine-Resistant

Canine Transmissible Venereal Tumor"

It described the case of a female dog in Uruguay with identical chemo-resistant circumstances as Cassie's but with a backside tumor nearly four times the size. This dog's tumor had been successfully dissolved with only three doses of Lomustine. The report's 'after' photograph showed that her humongous bulge had shrunk *to nothing*. Like Cassie's trial-and-error journey, this other dog's serendipitous remedy was not a clinical trial: it too was a shot in the dark out of desperation. Although the two cases were unconnected and occurred remarkably simultaneously, Cassie's past seven days of symptom decline seemed to be proving that our results would be exactly the same.

My heart soaring, I jumped to my feet with the long-awaited grant of a wish-come-true. As I danced around in high-octane glee, Cassie's wiggling Boxer butt joined her Hooman in the fun. We found it. We found *the cure*!

Just when that unshakable invader was ready to grow again, it was sent into oblivion by a super-charged chemical and the tenacious wagging of a puppy dog's tail.

SPRUNG

Spring is that time of year for chicks and bunnies and dripping Cadbury egg goo all over pastel-colored outfits. To the devout, it brings prayers over traditional meals and songs of re-birth. After a spell of interminable darkness, it is a time of brightness and joy.

Such was my heart as Cassie and I made the ninety-minute drive to spend Easter Saturday with Mom and her now long-time caregiver, my sister Mary. Regular phone calls with Mom over the past month had kept her informed on Cassie's *miracle cure* and I looked forward to sharing my daughter's newly regained energy with her.

It was amazing how quickly Cassie rebounded following the Lomustine chemotherapy. After the first pill, her tumor shrank to the size of a pea, the relief from which found my girl running jubilant zoomies in the backyard nearly non-stop. Her perineum bulge deflated noticeably plus she was ravenous, gaining back poundage with each week. Three Lomustine pills were originally prescribed - one every four weeks. However, her sustained good health, the success of the first dosage and the incredible results of her counterpart in Uruguay prompted me to beg for the interval to be shortened. Dr. Rambaud cleared Cassie's condition as being robust enough so Dr. Brignone approved the second wonder drug pill to go down her throat a week early.

Seventeen days later, we were on our way to the celebratory visit. Although I had tucked diapers, under pads and her pink-leopard overalls in the corner of the car's trunk out of habit (*just in case*) they remained there without retrieval. Cassie's symptoms were nonexistent and had begun their fade from memory. Entering the living room with no worries of carpet stains or contagion drip within nose-shot of little Corky, my sister's dog was a simple freedom I was just beginning to relish.

Mom was sitting in her favorite chair and Cassie bounded over for some Gramma sniffs and a kiss. I was dismayed at how gaunt Mom seemed as she gently reached out to return Cassie's affection. The two dogs had a guarded meet-and-greet and I could see the contagion-worried look on Mary's face as she supervised their re-acquaintance.

"She hasn't dripped in more than a month," I reassured her. Cassie headed straight to Corky's stash of stuffed toys, picked one and enthusiastically nudged me for a throw. Corky easily loped onto Mom's lap, finding a place of safety from this larger dog's energy while resuming his accustomed role as comfort animal. Mom's feeble hand began a familiar caress and her eyelids drooped.

"Do you want to take a nap, Mom?" I asked in a hushed tone. Cassie brushed by her blue recliner in a high-energy return for another toy toss down the hallway behind the chair rousing Mom a little.

"She's fine," Mary said, looking up from the kitchen-island cooktop as she prepared our dinner. "This is normal for her," she added with resignation.

"No… no… I'm awake," Mom said, then with a voice renewed by amazement she continued, "Cassie looks so normal! She's like a different dog than she was last time." I agreed, remembering how just last Christmas, our visit's activities were still limited by Cassie's chemo-induced lethargy and, of course, bloody discharge.

Mom strained to turn in her chair watching Cassie bound after the toy, a weak smile wrinkling her 102-year-old face. She asked how it happened. I didn't mind a re-telling of our little victories starting with how vincristine seemed to break up the mass making it pliable which allowed surgical removal of a chunk.

I could see that Mom's eyes were barely open and I wondered if my detailed recitation was taxing her. Mary, who had been listening as she basted the roast, refused to look at the photo of the de-bulked mass I held out from my phone gallery and instead surmised, "I bet she's more comfortable with that gone. I can't even imagine what that would have felt like… ugh…"

I continued the story about Lomustine, the Uruguay dog and Cassie's non-existent discharge but the conversation proceeded only between Mary and me. Mom was in slumber.

With a tone of worry I observed in a whisper, "Mom seems really out of it." We spoke a bit about Mom's mental state. "She usually is fine during our phone calls," I offered, "but not always. I hate it when she says, '*I wish God would just take me.*' I never know what to say in response."

Mary looked over at her with a sad face clearly displaying reluctant *acceptance*. From her many years as first Dad's, and now Mom's caregiver --- a time spent taking them to and from doctor appointments, filling prescriptions and providing comfort during their time

146

left --- Mary recognized the inevitable.

Wiping her hands, she came over to Mom and gently rubbing her thin shoulder said, "Dinner's almost ready, Mom. Do you want to eat at the table? Or shall I set up the tray tables here?"

Opening her eyes, Mom joined us again. "Let's eat at the table," she answered quietly.

"Yes, it's Easter!" I said and went to set the table.

Keeping a keen eye on her Mommie now headed to the yummy-smelling room and seeing that Corky was maintaining his place of honor on Mom's lap, Cassie plopped down next to his Gramma at the foot of the recliner. A lovely Madonna scene enveloped the blue easy chair.

While pulling out Mom's good dishes, I recalled a strikingly similar image. My never-ending Facebook scrolling had recently located photos of a very important person from Cassie's puppy days: her first caretaker, Anita. The dark-haired lady depicted in those on-line posts was the hooman who welcomed Cassie off the streets. This woman selflessly fostered 'Ciara' through that first bout of TVT taking her to those weeks of Facebook-friend-funded mange baths and the vincristine chemo treatments. In a chain-link fenced yard with meager supplies, Anita nursed the puppy back to health, socialized her with a pack of equally compromised street dogs and when cured, sent her north to find her *domicilio especial.*

I have the honor of being Cassie's fur-ever Mommie, but she was Ciara's Mom. Anita cared for my then *Ciara* just the same as my Mom had cared for me.

The Mother-Daughter relationship is a special attachment of care, created wholly chaste from that first undertaking then evolves with life's ups and downs. The bond, granted by a Higher Power or perhaps attained through serendipity, is directed nonetheless by instinct. It is bound by the mother's legacy of either manacles or satin bonnet strings. Though the pair may not always be in accord and the alliance oft-times fraught with tough-love, (be it life-changing, be it long-forgiven,) a daughter's soul is shaped by the role model which, I have come to know, transcends species.

Cassie was taught trust and resilience by Anita.

I learned loyalty and endurance from my Mom.

148

Mom passed away ten days after that last supper. She asked Mary to help her to bed just as we were leaving that evening and she never got up again. Mary, the youngest of her seven, eased Mom's way to Heaven, reversing the role of caregiver on behalf of her progeny.

My heart was heavy with the profound loss of my Mother. But I can't help wondering if, in His Mysterious Ways, God timed the trials with Cassie so that joys of her renewed health should somehow temper this anguished time of mourning to soften my soul as any mother would wish.

I am so very grateful to be able to have our final *Good-bye*. Blooms of geraniums, her favorite flower, spring forth in my garden now where Mom is at peace in her rightful place next to Dad's red rose, sweetening our Blessings.

WHERE CREDIT IS DUE

I so wanted to feel normal again. The ecstatic highs of Cassie's cure combined with grief-induced lows of Mom's loss had torn my psyche in two. I sorely missed my daily phone calls with Mom and had nearly forgotten that *sans tumor*, Cassie was a happy rescue puppy who adopted me as her hooman three years ago. Her rough-and-tumble beginnings on the street may have made her *extra* hardy indeed. The extraordinary rejuvenation was a heart-felt reminder.

An unprecedented chemo-therapy treatment called Lomustine had melted Cassie's sarcoma, yet after years of *treatment-shrinkage-regrowth-treatment-shrinkage-regrowth,* I maintained a germ of skepticism. During one of our post-tumor check-ups, I asked Dr. Rambaud to certify Cassie's remission in writing. I needed to read the printed words to convince myself.

It read:

Dear Ms. Mudge,

I examined Cassie today during her weekly acupuncture treatment. I could find no residual evidence of her vaginal TVT, meaning that she is now in remission. She is not contagious and poses no risk to other dogs....

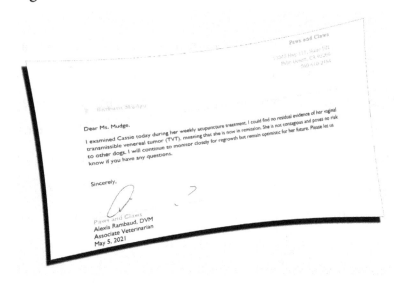

Paws and Claws
73343 Hwy 111, Suite 101
Palm Desert, CA 92260
760-610-2154

Barbaura Mudge

Dear Ms. Mudge,

I examined Cassie today during her weekly acupuncture treatment. I could find no residual evidence of her vaginal transmissible venereal tumor (TVT), meaning that she is now in remission. She is not contagious and poses no risk to other dogs. I will continue to monitor closely for regrowth but remain optimistic for her future. Please let us know if you have any questions.

Sincerely,

Paws and Claws
Alexis Rambaud, DVM
Associate Veterinarian
May 5, 2021

This signed prognosis became a document for our future.

As Cassie discovered long-abandoned toys in every household cranny, I found catharsis preparing my eulogy for Mom's mid-summer memorial service. The reminder of her life put to paper brought tear-stained smiles back to my face. Witnessing Cassie's zoomies run round and round the backyard pool, I dotted my Furringdomland group *shares* with happy exclamation marks.

Cassie's reawakened little woof-whine voice

joined in with the neighborhood dogs howling at far off sirens and warned the cats next door that she was back on duty. She's again at doggy day care, shadows her Mommie while in the garden and favors one particular patch of backyard sand for her contented naps.

As I watched her spirit, I grew more and more beholden to the people - from all around the world - who were responsible for her medical contributions as well as those extending much-needed emotional support to me. It was a gratitude that needed to be expressed beyond a simple *'Thank You.'* I was compelled to offer a grander gesture, if only for the locals. The joys of our *return to normal* deserved a Big Splash.

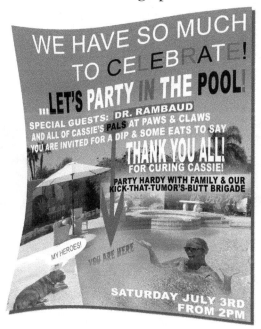

I believe that this celebratory cleansing served well to wash away my resentment for those who may have impeded Cassie's rightful destiny as a normal dog. I haven't really given them a second thought focusing instead on the more important matters of settling into a routine at last: active mornings followed by afternoon snoozes and plenty of cuddling by day's end.

Giving due credit to the scientists devoted to their research on Cassie's endowment, with high hopes we await breakthrough cancer discoveries benefitting canines and possibly even humankind.

Until then, Cassie and I will be here sharing a life unremarkable.

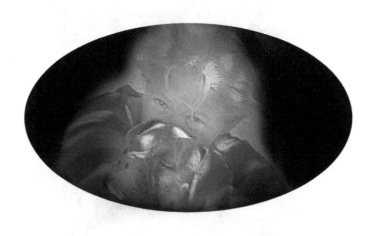

EPILOGUE

Our together smell is happy again.

Not like those many many sleeps ago when I licked you, never tasting your smile. Or when the tang of all those stings poofed from my fur and goo stink floated in the air. Or from the salty water that rolled from your eyes when I heard your sad.

That was long ago when the happy was gone.

The happy is back, tho. My tail wags now that our fur-ever smell has returned to what we made when first you held my face and I hugged you tight. We have our good mix again. An odor ours alone.

Our perfect scent.

The one that's easy to breathe.

The one made only by My Hooman and me.

CIARA

Exact birth unknown
perhaps September 2015
or maybe January 2016?

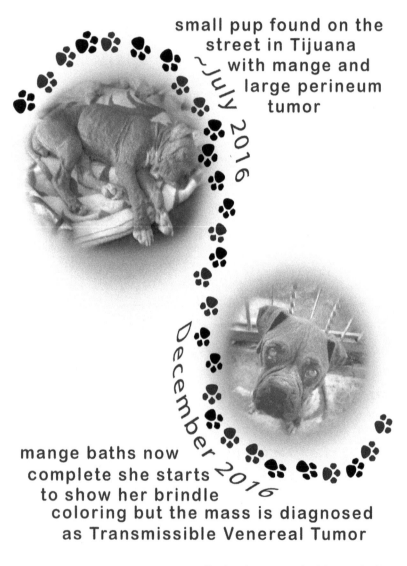

small pup found on the
street in Tijuana
~July 2016 with mange and
large perineum
tumor

December 2016

mange baths now
complete she starts
to show her brindle
coloring but the mass is diagnosed
as Transmissible Venereal Tumor

Early photos used with permission

CIARA

brave little girl
ready for her first
chemotherapy

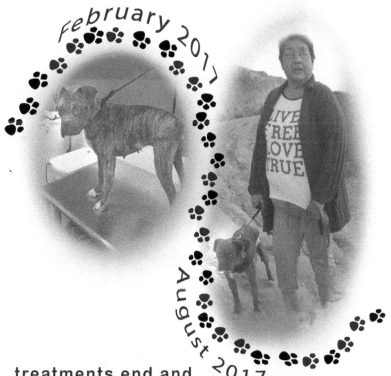

February 2017

August 2017

treatments end and
now "cured" of the TVT
she goes on a goodbye walk with
her hooman, Anita before traveling
to a new life in the USA

from Guardian Angel, Nancy Goodwin

APPENDIX

CASSIE

placed with West Coast Boxer Rescue September 2017

renamed "Cassie," a happy puppy first meets her fur-ever Hooman

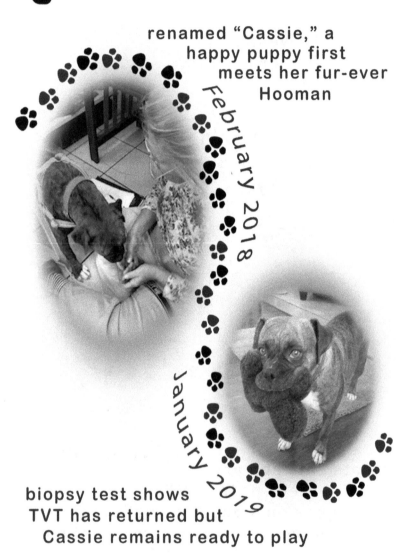

February 2018

January 2019

biopsy test shows TVT has returned but Cassie remains ready to play

CASSIE

August 2020

always keeps a toy
close by when chemo
side effects make
it hard to get
out of bed...

February 2021

yet fifty-one
chemos later and
she's still on her feet!

CASSIE

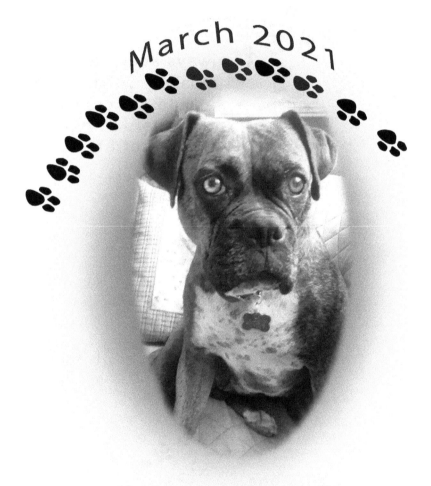

March 2021

unorthodox chemo, Lomustine
delivers the miracle cure and
puts the sparkle back in her eyes

CASSIE

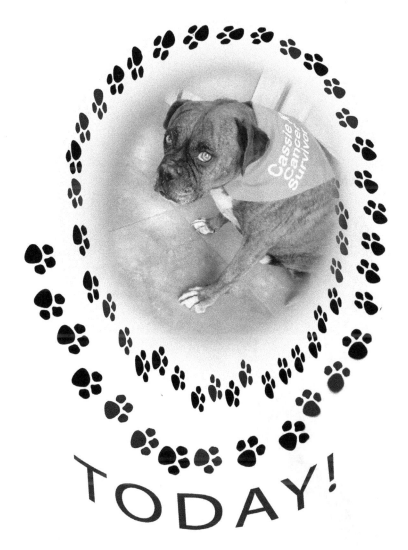

TODAY!

OUR PACK AT THE

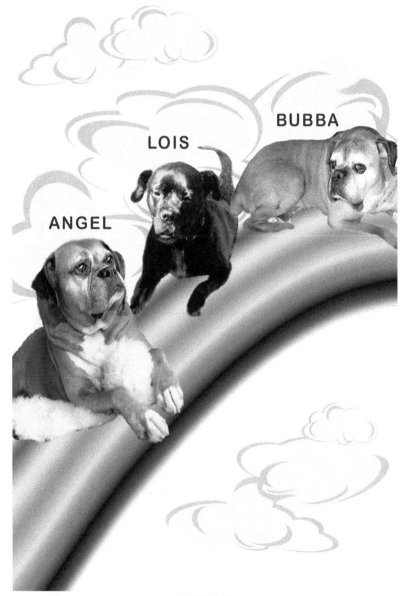

BUBBA

LOIS

ANGEL

RAINBOW BRIDGE

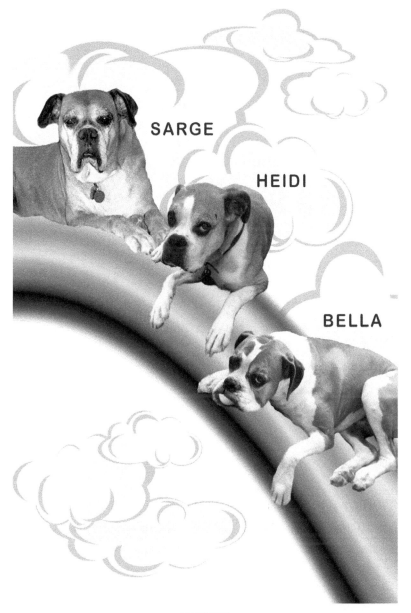

SARGE

HEIDI

BELLA

LINKS

West Coast Boxer Rescue

https://westcoastboxerrescue.org/

Boxer Rescue Los Angeles

https://boxer-rescue-la.com/

Dog Gone Tired Sanctuary & Rescue

http://www.doggonetiredsanctuary.com/

On Facebook:

Nancy Goodwin (Chez Nany)

https://www.facebook.com/AngelsTogetherForever

Furringdomland

https://www.facebook.com/groups/8018119987

My Hooman And Me

https://www.facebook.com/clubmudge2

ABOUT THE AUTHOR

BARBARA A. MUDGE

An accomplished writer of short-form prose adaptations of produced works, Barbara's words have had international audiences in marketing and promotion fields for more than forty years. Her career in the motion picture industry includes extensive film sales plus executive producer credits and screenplay consultation at every budget level.

Barbara's life-long affinity for the power of true stories inspired MY HOOMAN AND ME. Throughout her arduous caretaking of Cassie, Barbara sought help of any kind but found little. She hopes that this *waggling tale* may serve others facing the similar and reveal the remarkable serendipity of their story.

Her other mission in its writing is to accompany the science of the Cambridge Veterinarian Group's research results when completed with a more personal look at Cassie's life.

Alongside healthy wigglebutt Cassie, Barbara resides in the Coachella Valley in Southern California where she enjoys creative landscaping, crosswords in ink and the occasional round of golf.